Also by Valerie Davis Raskin, M.D.

When Words Are Not Enough: The Women's Prescription for Depression and Anxiety
This Isn't What I Expected: Recognizing and Recovering from Postpartum Depression (with Karen Kleinman)

GREAT SEX *for* MOMS

Ten Steps to Nurturing
Passion While Raising Kids

VALERIE DAVIS RASKIN, M.D.

A Fireside Book
Published by Simon & Schuster New York London Toronto Sydney Singapore

FIRESIDE

Rockefeller Center
1230 Avenue of the Americas
New York, NY 10020

Copyright © 2002 by Valerie Davis Raskin

FIRESIDE and colophon are registered trademarks
of Simon & Schuster, Inc.

For information about special discounts for bulk purchases,
please contact Simon & Schuster Special Sales:
1-800-456-6798 or business@simonandschuster.com

Designed by Bonni Leon-Berman
Manufactured in the United States of America

10 9 8 7 6 5 4 3 2 1

Library of Congress Cataloging-in-Publication Data

Raskin, Valerie D.
    Great sex for moms : ten steps to nurturing passion while raising kids / Valerie
Davis Raskin.
    p. cm.
Includes bibliographical references.
    1. Sex instruction for women. 2. Mothers—Sexual behavior. 3. Parenting. I. Title.
HQ46.R37 2002
613.9'07'1—dc21   2001057622
ISBN 0-7432-1265-7

Contents

Conclusion
Consolidating Change 223

Introduction

Most of us think everyone else has a better sex life.

We may be doctors or patients, stay-at-home moms or utilizers of daycare, firefighters or librarians. Whether we've been married for decades or are single moms, moms for days or for decades, most of us think everyone else is enjoying a more erotic, pleasurable, intimate—you fill in the blank—sex life.

If we're moms, we're convinced of it.

We imagine that our best friend, our sister, the nurse down the block, the lady at the supermarket checkout, and our partner's last girlfriend know no woe when it comes to libido.

In the absence of information, we buy into the myths. We believe that most women climax during conventional intercourse.

They don't.

We believe that most married couples make love three times a week.

Not true.

We believe that sex drive should come back when you stop breast-feeding.

It doesn't.

We believe that our partners obsess about our bodies as much as we do.

Thank goodness, they don't.

We believe that sexuality is instinctual, and that if the thrill is gone, it won't come back.

It most certainly can.

Along with our mistaken beliefs about everyone else's sex life, we assume that we are powerless to change our sexual relationship. We are often afraid that the only solutions will involve a sex therapist with a secret treasure chest in the back office, filled with studded black leather collars, French maid costumes, plastic purple things that require batteries, and videos you can't find at Blockbuster.

Most likely, you remember when sex was great: before kids. You may even look forward again to great sex, in the *very* distant future. As far as the present goes, though, chances are that you've given up. You are convinced that restoring passion to your sex life means becoming Scandinavian, igniting an affair, or learning Houdini-like contortions.

I hope to change your mind.

You *can* have a good sex life and raise children. You may believe that you're simply too tired or too busy for sex, but even exhausted moms can have energy tucked away for sex. I will show you how. And if you think you're too shy to improve your sexual relationship, I'll give you a cure for self-consciousness.

How can I help? What makes me someone you should trust? I can tell you this: I never intended to be a doctor who specializes in sex. In fact, I'm still hoping my mother doesn't find out. But in the years I've been practicing psychotherapy, and in the years I've been a mom, I've come to understand how easily passion withers, how guilty and alone so many women feel about their sexual indifference, and how quickly emotional disconnection can follow sexual disconnection in a marriage. I've also learned that ignoring the problem—tempting as that is—doesn't make it go away.

As a psychiatrist, I focus on treating women with reproductive-related problems, such as postpartum depression, panic disorder in pregnancy, and PMS (premenstrual syndrome). Considering where babies come from, I have more than my share of patients who recently have had sex, and many more who plan to have, or at least enjoy, sex once the kids leave for college.

I hear my postpartum patients wish they'd never have to have sex again. I hear women feeling guilty, certain their husbands got cheated in the karma lottery when they got stuck with them, instead of all those other women who climax at the mere thought of intercourse. I hear how love and romance fade into the background of carpools, laundry, and bake sales. I hear about how years of Doing It the same way gets old. I hear about kids who barge into the parental bedroom, and kids who drain all energy, sexual and otherwise. I hear about husbands who don't ever help with the housework but expect sex on demand. I hear about the intricacies of sexual life as a single parent. I hear about how teenagers never go to sleep, and how teenagers who cannot hear the alarm clock when it's time to get up for school have an uncanny radar for the hushed sounds behind closed doors that just might indicate parental romance.

I also hear about the imagined great sex life of others: the sister who went on a second honeymoon to the Caribbean and claimed she had sex 24-7, the friend who went to New Orleans with her husband for a weekend without the kids and never left the hotel, the neighbor who accidentally on purpose keeps her window open so that everyone knows what a stud her husband is.

But I hear all this only when I ask.

It puzzled me at first that moms would talk about sex only when pressed, even in therapy. Why were moms holding back? The lightbulb went off when a patient told me that I couldn't understand her sexual problem with her husband because my own sex life was, undoubtedly, fantastic. Patients' idealization is nothing new to a therapist, but this one seemed especially poignant. A patient who understood that as a fellow mom, I know as well she does the truth behind the Hallmark version of motherhood, simply couldn't imagine that I knew this dark little secret of motherhood, too. She believed that compared to others, her bedroom was uniquely awkward, tense and boring.

While we laugh about men anxiously comparing penis size, it turns out that we women make comparisons, too. Trained since about fifth grade to notice who's prettier, smarter, thinner, or more popular, as adults we women often have deep imagined sexual shortcomings, too. We think our bedroom credentials are so woefully inadequate that we're hopeless. By comparison to the "in-crowd," we feel deficient.

There is great news here: You aren't the only one. Even better news: You can have great sex again, even as a great mom. It isn't one or the other. Indeed, you *must* address the sexual blahs. Great sex is an important aspect of a happy relationship, and happy parents are the cornerstones of happy families.

The solutions I've discovered in the years I've practiced medicine are simple steps that real-world moms can do. But not so fast. Before tackling the Ten Steps to Nurturing Passion, I want you to get clear about the things standing in the way. Think of it this way: When you take your car to the shop for a tune-up, your mechanic runs some tests to see how the engine is running, even if you think you already know what needs attention. Likewise, a careful and honest exploration of the sexual issues in your life will get you headed in the right direction.

Why bother? Why not jump ahead to the solutions? Most important, the proper self-diagnosis almost always makes you feel better about yourself. If you have emotional or sexual issues, it's reassuring to know that your problems are commonplace. It's ever so heartening to know that others have overcome similar challenges. What a relief to discover that no one is to blame, that neither you nor your husband belongs to the Hall of Shame. How encouraging it is to know that Personally and Hopelessly Defective is the wrong diagnosis.

It's not your fault. It's not his fault.

While there are many things that a mother can do to enhance her sexuality, the prerequisite is to stop feeling guilty. Blaming yourself, feeling inadequate, feeling sorry for the poor, unfortunate husband who got stuck with you gets in the way of making changes. Blaming him also puts up roadblocks. Guilt and anger make poor bedfellows. Great sex starts with good self-esteem and mutual regard.

It isn't your fault that you're tired all the time. It isn't his fault that he wants to make love even when you're tired. It isn't your child's fault that her sleeping patterns are wreaking havoc on your sexual relationship. It isn't your husband's fault that he doesn't know how to touch you in ways that are more enjoyable. It isn't your fault that you haven't ever told him how you wish to be touched. It isn't your fault that society tries to tell you that everyone else in the world has mind-blowing sex night after night.

For a society with nearly naked women on billboards, Victoria's Secret at every mall, and MTV videos that would cause our grandmothers to roll over in their graves, we're actually terribly inhibited sexually when it comes to face-to-face conversation about sexuality with a sexual partner. Think of how many couples see R-rated movies together, with explicit images of sexuality, but never, ever talk about their own sexual relationship. We're frozen by our sense of inadequacy, afraid that speaking up will only point out the ways we fail to measure up. Your male partner likely has the same worry, and perhaps you are afraid to speak up for fear that he'll feel criticized or emasculated.

Throughout this book, I'll be encouraging you to find your voice sexually. I understand that this seems impossible, but I also know that you can do it. I know that if it were easy for you, you'd have done so ages ago. I promise to help, to give you specific tools and specific words to use.

I believe that if you want a better sexual relationship, so does your partner. I also believe that books that make extravagant promises about quick fixes and cosmic orgasms aren't for you. In fact, these outrageous myths ("Earth-shattering climaxes in ten seconds a day") actually make you feel worse. It's like picking up a book that tells you how to be the perfect mother: It only makes you feel more deficient to be told that you ought to be able to charm your two-year-old out of a temper tantrum, or that perfect moms don't ever raise their voices at their teenagers.

I believe that any woman can experience an orgasm, if she's comfortable with what it takes to get there. I do believe that any woman can learn to talk more openly about her body and her sexual needs with her husband. I believe that boring sex can be made interesting. I don't believe in perfect sex, any more than I believe in perfect mothers.

I do believe in good-enough mothers and great sex.

This book will tell you about the realities, about what sex in other people's bedrooms is really like. It will help you see yourself more realistically, and take courage from the fact that you are not alone in the sexual rut of motherhood. It will give you practical words to use with your partner. It will give you simple ideas that can enhance the romance and intimacy of sexuality, without pushing you beyond the limits of your own comfort.

The Ten Steps to Nurturing Passion While Raising Kids are much like those you would use to develop any new skill or revisit a neglected one. If you used to knit but no longer do, if you always meant to learn a new language but haven't gotten around to it, if you think you might take up tae kwon do one of these days when you find the time, you know what it's going to take. You have to make the decision, commit the necessary time and space, get the right tools, persevere, and tolerate the first few awkward attempts.

So too with overcoming the sexual blahs. First, you have to establish priorities that support the values of sexuality, self-care, and self-regard. I will steer you toward making better choices for yourself. I will teach you to quiet the inner voice that constantly murmurs "You can't." Next, you will need to acquire new skills. I'll facilitate your journey, as you cultivate your sensual mind, attention, confidence, and knowledge. Finally, I'll ask you to set these skills in motion, expanding just beyond the too-comfortable zone.

The major human sex organ is above the neck. That's a blessing and a curse. Sexual boredom, inertia, fatigue, fear, alienation, and negative cultural scripts are in the mind. It usually isn't anything physiologically related to motherhood. Because the obstacles to great sex are often mental, the good news is that you can infuse your sexuality with excitement, spirit, energy, confidence, connection, and self-affirmation. Indeed, this book is about making small changes with substantial benefits. It's about everyday women enhancing their sex lives. It's about ordinary mothers overcoming ordinary sexual problems.

I'll suggest that what goes on in your mind, what goes on in your romantic relationship, what goes on in your daily life affects your sexuality as a mother. Loving mothers pay attention to their sex lives. Families are more threatened by sexual blahs than by parents who sneak off for a weekend alone. I'll encourage you to keep an open mind. After all, you already have all that you need to enjoy an honest, loving, safe, mature, pleasurable, and emotionally gratifying sexual relationship.

The
Diagnosis

The Four Obstacles to
GREAT SEX for MOMS

Motherhood and sex have a lot in common. When they're great, they're really great. When they're monotonous, or downright disagreeable, you can be sure that most people are *not* going to admit it. Culturally, when it comes to sex and motherhood, we amplify the good while pretending the bad doesn't exist. This conspiracy of silence adds insult to injury: If it's so good for others, it's awfully tempting to blame oneself for one's troubles.

But here's the truth: It's not so great for everyone else. If you're struggling with sexuality and motherhood, take comfort in knowing that many share your plight. There are plenty of obstacles to great sex and many understandable reasons that mothers put off nurturing sexuality.

The next few chapters will help you substitute a more accurate and forgiving diagnosis than "hopeless" or "helpless." Expect to recognize elements of inertia and denial in your own self-assessment. They're that prevalent. Motherhood is a never-ending hundred-yard dash, and minimizing and overlooking unmet challenges is inevitable. But as inviting as a little what-you-don't-admit-can't-hurt-you can be, it's time to reassess priorities and to rebalance.

While most mothers experience bouts of running on empty, some face the very serious challenge of excessive maternal sacrifice. These mothers are so massively exhausted that unless they slay the demon of giving too much, sex will remain a chore. Be sure to read this chapter if you struggle with perfectionism.

Sexual issues actually may be relationship issues in disguise. If you are having significant marital problems, of course you will have sexual issues. It will not be useful to isolate sexual disinterest as the problem when the accurate diagnosis is a troubled marriage. Use this chapter to help you discern whether sexual disconnection is actually due to marital disconnection.

Finally, a word of caution. Consider whether something other than the emotional challenges of raising kids is ruining your sex life. The obstacles described here and the Ten Steps to Nurturing Passion are directed at the reader who used to find sex enjoyable before kids. If lovemaking has never been remotely pleasurable, you may need a different approach. Alternatively, if you have had a very sudden or complete drop in all sexual thoughts, fantasies, or interest, you may have a physiological cause, such as hormone imbalance or medication side effects. Be sure to consider a physical component. Sexual dysfunction and physiological causes of low libido are described in Step Ten and Appendix B. A careful medical history and physical examination by your personal physician is an excellent place to start before tackling the emotional solutions described in this book.

The First Obstacle: Reality

Having Great Sex as a Mom Is Challenging

> "Almost no attention has been paid . . . to the sexual needs, desires or experiences of women once they make the transition to motherhood."
>
> —Judith C. Daniluk, *Women's Sexuality Across the Lifespan*

- Phases of family life have a predictable impact on mothers' sexuality.
- You must not surrender to the forces that conspire to ruin your sex life.
- Great sex is worth the effort.

If you're a mother, at some time in your life—maybe many times—you haven't had the energy for making love. If you're a mother, chances are good that you have a pretty full plate, one that just doesn't seem to have room for sex. Making matters worse, you probably have much less interest than your husband,[1] who simply doesn't ever seem too tired.

Sex may have become a burden, or you may have found yourself participating with your mind on other things. You may still make love as often as you did before the kids, but not with the enjoyment you once had. If you're making love out of guilt or a sense of obligation, you may rather just get it over with, not really valuing your own pleasure and counting the minutes until he's "done."

---

[1] Here and throughout this book, substitute whatever word fits for you: partner, boyfriend, lover.

Perhaps from time to time, you wistfully remember those magical days when you used to crave sex, days when once wasn't enough. You may remember thinking that the stereotype about women never wanting sex once they get married would never apply to you. You may remember a time when *you* were the one who started things rolling.

You may be wondering if something is physically wrong. Do you need hormones? Did something get damaged during childbirth? You may blame menopause, even if you're in your thirties. You may wonder if something you're taking is killing your libido, or if there isn't something you could take to get it back. Many of my patients wish something were wrong physically, because then they'd feel less guilty!

Am I the Only One?

Having great sex as a mom is a challenge shared by millions of women. For most, the damaging effects of child rearing are far less physical than emotional. Moms don't usually talk much with girlfriends about the actual details of sex, and almost never about sexual pleasure. That means that although you may have laughed together about how you wished your obstetrician would give you the medical equivalent of a note for the principal excusing you from sex, you almost certainly don't talk about the quality of your sex lives.

I bet that you don't know whether your best friend has orgasms or how often she makes love with her husband. I bet she doesn't know whether your husband is the best lover you've ever been with or the worst. I bet you don't know whether she thinks oral sex is fantastic or vulgar. Sharing the specifics of your sex life may simply be taboo, or it may feel like a betrayal of the intimacy you share with your husband.

If you have talked, chances are that you found that your best friend also noticed that passion waned somewhere along the path of motherhood. If you have talked together, you may have wondered whether it happens to every woman, and you may have questioned whether things will ever be like they used to be.

If you know you're not the only one, you're right. Sexual mismatches between husbands and wives, or between single mothers and their partners, are very common. And while it is common for healthy women and men alike to make love well into their grandparent and great-grandparent years, it's also common for mothers actively raising children to have less interest in sex than their partners do.

- One third of women between the ages of 18 and 59 report a lack of sexual desire.
- Low sexual desire is the most common reason individuals seek treatment for sexual problems.

"Once the Kids Are . . ."

You can complete this sentence countless ways. Once the kids are sleeping through the night, I'll want to make love again. Once the kids are in school, I won't be too tired for sex. Once the kids go to camp, our sex life will flourish again. Once the kids start high school, we'll have Saturday nights to ourselves again. Once the kids go to college, things will be just like they used to be.

Unfortunately, there isn't a stage of active motherhood that doesn't have the potential to annihilate your sex life. Twenty years is a long time to give up an enjoyable sex life, and, unfortunately, many marriages are threatened by sexual incompatibility. Even if you're sure that your marriage isn't at risk, it's a high price to pay for the pleasure of having children. Fortunately, you can make small but meaningful changes that will bring the spark back, and you don't have to—and shouldn't—keep putting your sexual pleasure on the back burner.

First, let's look at reality. Reviewing the concrete obstacles specific to the stages of raising kids is an important aspect of making an accurate self-assessment.

Mothers of Infants

For many mothers, the first encounter with low sex drive follows childbirth. The obstetrician typically blesses resumption of intercourse at four to six weeks after delivery, a time that virtually always seems like forever to dads and ridiculously soon for moms.

Babies are exhausting, and sleepless night after sleepless night drains all energy, sexual or otherwise. Other factors that contribute to low sex drive after childbirth include soreness (especially if there are lacerations or stitches), recovery from surgery (cesarean section), anemia (which can be determined by a simple blood test), and hormone changes (especially if you're breast-feeding).

Even when the physical healing is underway, libido is usually quite low for up to a year after childbirth because physical energy is so scarce. Most new mothers feel like they operate on autopilot, never getting ahead of the mountain of chores. Even easy babies are hard at times and can wear you out when they are teething, colicky, or over-tired. Even when the father handles some of the night feedings, the ultimate responsibility is usually the mother's, especially during the early months.

Breast-feeding kills libido, a particular irony since many husbands find that seeing their wives nurturing a baby in this way is very arousing. Some of it's a chemical problem. When functioning as usual, the ovaries make a small amount of testosterone, which contributes to sex drive (and helps explain one of the differences between the male and female libido). Breast-feeding suppresses the ovarian production of testosterone, and what little interest might have been there is reduced even further.

But the negative impact breast-feeding has on sex drive isn't just chemical. Many women describe feeling completely businesslike about their bodies. As Cindy said, "Once you whip your breast out in the grocery store line to soothe a screaming baby, it loses all sensual significance." Others feel that the physical depletion of breast-feeding is so overwhelming that it literally drains all their other physical aspects. One mother said, "I love nursing, but after a day of it, my body wants some time for itself." Other nursing moms feel that the act of nursing is so enjoyable that they just don't have the same need to be touched affectionately.

Postpartum depression, a condition experienced by one in three mothers, further depletes sexual interest. Along with crying spells, low self-esteem, anxiety attacks, and sleeplessness even when the baby sleeps, low libido is a symptom of depression. Making matters worse, most of the antidepressants prescribed for postpartum depression (those that increase serotonin; e.g., Prozac, Zoloft, Paxil, Luvox, Effexor, Celexa, Anafranil) have low libido and inability to climax as common side effects.[2]

---

[2] If you are suffering from postpartum depression, it is necessary to address this issue first. Don't isolate the sexual symptom and don't dismiss postpartum depression as "just baby blues." For more information, see Karen Kleinman and Valerie Davis Raskin, *This Isn't What I Expected: Overcoming Postpartum Depression* (New York: Bantam, 1994).

- Two thirds of women report decreased sexual frequency after kids are born.
- By four months postpartum, one fifth of new parents have not resumed lovemaking.
- At six months after the birth of a first child, two thirds of women report sexual problems.

Mothers of Toddlers and Preschoolers

During the first year after childbirth, many couples believe that once they get some sleep, things will get back to normal. It is often a rude surprise to discover that maternal demands during the toddler and preschool years are such that sexual energy remains low. From doing laundry to cajoling a two-year-old out of a temper tantrum, a mother's seemingly endless list of tasks can wear down her libido.

In fact, some mothers feel most drained during the preschool years. At least babies nap often and are easier to keep safe than a two-year-old who climbs furniture, goes for the electric outlets, and tries to eat the dog food. Like mothers of babies, women with young children feel someone at their bodies all day long. It's natural and understandable to want some space, privacy, and recovery time. Sleep is not predictable yet, as anything from an ear infection to nightmares can interrupt lovemaking and prevent a couple from having time that they can count on for themselves.

Another sexual stressor during this phase is lengthy or difficult bedtime rituals, and certain methods of getting children of this age to go to sleep. After giving a bath (which may have included forced hair washing), picking out pajamas, getting a bedtime snack, locating the special blanket or mandatory stuffed animal that got stuck behind the couch, reading "just one more" story, and rubbing a child's back, many mothers either fall asleep as their preschoolers do or crawl bleary-eyed into their own beds.

Although postpartum depression is increasingly recognized, it turns out that there is another big secret about motherhood and depression: The period of highest risk for clinical depression among mothers is during the toddler years. This is an especially vulnerable time for stay-at-home mothers, but none is immune. Review the symptoms of depression in Step Ten (on page 209), and stop putting off getting help for yourself if this is a problem you're experiencing.

- Almost 1 in 10 couples are not sexually active by their child's first birthday.
- At one year postpartum, couples who have resumed love-making usually have sex once per week.

Mothers of Elementary-Age Children

Although the kids are in school all day, many mothers are disappointed to find that they still don't have the libido they once had. But why not? First, many women take advantage of this new freedom to take on new projects or resume employment. Going back to college or graduate school, heading up the school parent-teacher organization, increasing from part-time to full-time work, or changing from an in-home nanny to a day care center quickly fills up the schedule. Suddenly things seem more, rather than less, hectic.

Children's lives are often busier, too. Kids don't drive themselves to play dates, dance classes, piano lessons, soccer practice, Boy Scouts, religious school, and basketball clubs. Many mothers have to load the younger kids in the car, too, each time any child has an activity. If your husband hasn't spent an afternoon getting a couple of children organized and ready to go at a moment's notice, then killed a half hour with a bored sibling or two waiting in the car during a flute lesson, run into the gas station for milk on the way home, and rushed right in to get dinner and homework started, he might not understand why you feel so exhausted at the end of the day.

Mothers of Teenagers

Privacy is the big issue when you have teenagers, many of whom view a closed bedroom door as an open invitation. The same child who insists that her bedroom is her private domain won't hesitate to barge right in when she wants or needs something from you.

In addition, the sleep cycles of teens usually interfere with parental privacy. Teens typically go to sleep around the same time you do, and you can be sure that they can stay up later than you can on weekends and holidays. Many parents hesitate to make love for fear that their kids will hear them or interrupt by banging on the locked door.

Sometimes teens are intruding because they're in the normal self-absorption of adolescence. It simply doesn't occur to them that you have or want a life of your own, sexual or otherwise. Other adolescents are struggling with issues of their own emerging sexuality, and it's not a coincidence that every time you lock your door, a kid suddenly materializes from nowhere. They don't want to think about you Doing It, and they make sure you cannot! This is especially common for single mothers, whose teenagers may have mixed feelings about the idea of a new man in Mom's life, including jealousy, anxiety, fear of being loved less, or ongoing wishes that you and their father would get back together.

Mixed Phases

Of course, if you have more than one child, your children may be in different phases. Some nights, the younger child wakes up minutes after the older one falls back to sleep. Other families describe weeks of illness circulating through the family. Just when you can stop the midnight dose for Tylenol for the child who brought home strep throat, it's your turn, and then your husband's turn to be ill. Who has the energy for sex?

Blended families may have his teen, her school-age kids, and their baby, or other configurations of widely spaced developmental stages. Such families also may have the added stress mentioned previously, of kids who subconsciously don't want you to have a new sex life.

Overcoming Inertia

If you rarely have the energy for making love, you may be so bogged down that you can't imagine trying to tackle the entire problem. If sex is too much on a specific evening, the prospect of addressing the larger problem may seem overwhelming.

I wish there were a shortcut, the sexual equivalent of beautiful abs in just minutes a day. Of course, you already know there isn't any such quick fix. It will take effort and attention. I acknowledge that this is tough. Why should you put forth the effort? Why try? Because great sex energizes rather than depletes you. Remember that sex, like motherhood, is really great when it's great. In a great sexual relationship after children, sex:

- communicates love and affection.
- soothes, comforts, and relaxes.

- bridges gaps when inevitable relationship conflict flares.
- affirms one's value.
- relieves stress outside and inside of marriage.
- is playful.
- enhances and is enhanced by emotional closeness.
- reminds you that you're "more than a mommy."
- delineates what is unique in marriage. It is what makes a couple more than best friends, more than business colleagues in an economic partnership, more than coparents.

Affirmation

"... sexual intimacy is something most couples will work at and refine throughout their married life ... wonderful things can happen."

—Stephen E. Lamb and Douglas E. Brinley, *Between Husband and Wife*

The Second Obstacle: Denial

Ignoring Boring Sex Is Tempting

> "Our biggest problem as human beings is not knowing that we don't know."
>
> —Virginia Satir

- If you think that something isn't right sexually, trust your instincts. You're probably right.
- If your husband thinks that something isn't right sexually, believe him. He's probably right.
- It takes two people to create sexual difficulties in a relationship. Be very skeptical of being labeled the "dysfunctional one."
- Denial enables small sexual problems to grow. Overcoming denial is the first step in reestablishing intimacy.

Perhaps you understand how Dana feels:

"At night, when my husband starts to touch me in that way that I know means he wants sex, I cringe inside. I really love him, but I could live without sex for at least a year, maybe a decade. After I've spent my days chasing two preschoolers, used nap time to pay bills, sat through excruciating reruns of *Barney* and *The Big Comfy Couch,* failed at keeping my two-year-old from changing outfits fourteen times before lunch, cleaned up after my four-year-old drew on the bathroom wallpaper, and almost cried when Lizzie took her boots and mittens off just when I finally got them on Jack, the last thing on my mind is sex. Truthfully, when my husband puts his hands on me, I feel like it's just one more person who wants something from me.

"It seems like I always blame the kids, but the truth is, I'm just as tired on the days I go into the office. Whether it's work or home, sometimes I think the whole world has a problem that I'm supposed to fix.

"I know he's upset that I say no so often when he wants to have sex. Part of me thinks he just won't grow up, that he's trying to pretend that he's still twenty. I want to say, 'Well, duh? What did you think it was going to be like having two little kids? Like, get real, welcome to Parenthood 101.' Another part of me thinks that he must be the unluckiest guy on the planet, because maybe there is something wrong with me. Is it normal for sex to be right up there with writing quarterly reports? Won't this get better when the kids are older?"

—*Dana, mother of Lizzie, two, and Jack, four*

When mothers ask me "what's normal" about sex after children, usually they mean, "How often is everyone else doing it?" If I could get away with writing about sexuality without answering the "how often" question, I surely would! It's a classic catch-22 question: There isn't an answer that is going to be remotely reassuring.

Women ask "How often?" for a few reasons. One is that they have a husband who is pressuring them to make love more often, and they're struggling with a sense of shame or failure. Another is that they are looking for support to feel more comfortable saying "not tonight." Occasionally, a woman asking the question is worried that her husband isn't sufficiently attracted to her. In all cases, the question indicates that something isn't right sexually.

If sex is enjoyable, interesting, and reflective of a couple's emotional intimacy, frequency isn't a very big issue. A couple with a strong physical connection isn't thinking comparatively. Anyone who feels that they have enough—whether it's material possessions or spiritual and emotional resources—isn't looking around to see what everyone else has.

Frequency is about as meaningful as penis size. Because I know that couples who make love every day can have an atrocious lack of intimacy, just as couples who make love once or twice a month can have a fantastic sexual relationship, my framework for sexuality emphasizes quality rather than quantity. In my system, great sex is characterized by communication, courage, caring, and connection. Pleasure naturally follows.

If either member of the couple is spending much time wondering about other people's sex lives, something is wrong. Often, as is true for Dana and her husband, both partners know that things have changed. They're both hoping it's nothing serious that time won't fix. Dana minimizes the problem by telling herself, "It just comes with the territory." She's moving toward recognizing the seriousness of the sexual disconnection, and as she does, she looks for an explanation: Is it the kids? The job? Is her husband oversexed? She's right not to blame herself. Unfortunately, insisting that there must be a single malfunction in need of a simple fix is itself a fancy form of denial.

Beyond "Dysfunction"

In this book, I will de-emphasize the concept of "sexual dysfunction." This term has some usefulness, especially in gathering statistics that let the public know that sexual unhappiness, despite cultural myths to the contrary, is epidemic in America. I welcome any term that helps a woman understand that she (or her partner) isn't the only one.

But I have some serious concerns about the term "sexual dysfunction," and you won't see it used much in this book.[1] If you can define "sexual dysfunction," you ought to be able to define "sexual function," but, aside from making babies, few of us would agree about what that is. Is it simply a matter of plumbing and electrical impulses working? Definitely not! Do you have to have cosmic orgasms night after night to have normal sexual functioning? No again.

The biggest problem with the term "sexual dysfunction" is that it points a finger at one member of the couple. I'll use terms such as "sexual difficulties" and "sexual issues" throughout this book, because sexuality is a relational issue, and good sex is a couple issue, not an individual issue. I see too many women who don't have much sex drive and who have labeled themselves or have been labeled as "dysfunctional." This label implies that low sex drive is a disease or defect within the individual woman. Labeling one member is really a form of denial, one that misses the big picture. Chances are that a sexually disinterested woman has a partner who is neglecting her, taking her for granted, criticizing her, rushing her in bed, dominating her, or in some way contributing to the problem.

"Dysfunction" implies that a sexual organ isn't working, and I believe that sexual issues for mothers are rarely problems of the pelvis.

Defining "good" sexual functioning strikes me as being a lot like defining happiness: If you have it, you know it. If you don't have it, no one can tell you that you do. If your instinct tells you that you have a sexual issue in your life, believe yourself. If your husband is

---

[1] For more information about medical descriptions of sexual dysfunction, see Appendix B: Sexual Dysfunction (Glossary of Terms).

telling you that he has a sexual issue, believe him, and understand that if he has an issue, so do you.

Overcoming Denial

While it might seem obvious that you should believe your instincts if you think something is wrong sexually, it's not that easy. Couples experiencing sexual difficulties always go through a period of denial.

Having children allows mothers (and fathers) to deny even longer than others, because their exhaustion is so very understandable. If either partner voices a sexual concern, one or both can immediately blame things on the children, who provide an easy excuse for not addressing the issue. It's easy to assume a helpless posture: If it's all the kids' fault, there's nothing parents can do until the kids are grown. Forget it!

Wait, aren't I saying that raising children has a huge negative impact on their parents' sex lives? Yes, of course. But that's not the whole story. It is a lot like hay fever: There is ragweed in the air everywhere, but only certain people sneeze every spring and summer. Kids are like a ragweed invasion. If there is any vulnerability in the sexual relationship, things go downhill rapidly. Some people sneeze with a little ragweed, others need to stick their heads in a pile of it to get symptoms. Symptoms of sexual blahs may show up under minimal "kid stress," or they may not appear until the child-related issues are overwhelming all aspects of parents' lives. Some couples need major work to overcome the sexual blahs, while others can overcome the difficulties with a little tune-up. But neither type of couple can fix things if one member chooses to pretend nothing is wrong.

In psychotherapy, one of the key principles is that honesty is the best policy. A truthful narrative, however painful, is always better than denial. For example, if you're in a difficult marriage, it's more pleasant to believe that you've been victimized by your spouse; that it's all his fault; that you've done everything possible to make it work, but he just won't stop doing that thing he keeps doing. The problem is that you can't do anything about that, and the price of the narrative that protects your ego also keeps you stuck.

The truth—perhaps that you chose him precisely because he does that thing he keeps doing and you have some unresolved issues around that thing—is the only path to freedom for both of you. True, rewriting the story may smart a little. If your story has been that children and above-average sex are mutually exclusive, rewriting the story may be a bit rocky. Ultimately, however, it will be worth the pain.

If you have been denying sexual problems in your marriage, you are undoubtedly trying to protect yourself from something alarming. Denial is a natural defense against the fear of opening Pandora's box. Denying intimacy issues is like having weeds in a corner of the garden. Even if you ignore them, they're still there. After a couple of months of ignoring them, the weeds are higher. Eventually, they creep into other areas of the garden, and sections of the yard that were perfectly fine go bad. After a few years, the weeds have spread so much that you can't even recognize the old garden. How much easier it would have been to remove the early weeds.

Am I suggesting that divorce—getting a whole new plot of land— is inevitable if you don't have a strong sexual relationship? Absolutely not. Do I think sexual difficulties contribute to divorce? Definitely. You know the brutal statistics: One in two marriages fail, and the numbers are even worse for second marriages. There is a cultural message making the rounds that we're "serial monogamists," incorrectly hardwired for maintaining sexual intimacy with just one person for the long haul. In such a system, extramarital affairs can be seen as biological phenomena, as if people had inevitable sexual urges to wander. I disagree.

Troubled marriages can cause bad sex, and trouble in marriage causes affairs, not vice versa. People enter affairs because they're unhappy and seeking affirmation, companionship, and comfort in both the emotional and the sexual arenas. Sexual blahs are not evolutionary destiny, and an exciting new sexual partner is not the evolutionary fix. You can remain sexually and emotionally connected for your lifetime with one partner, but it takes thought and work.

To do so, you need to recognize two issues that have nothing to do with divorce. First, survival isn't good enough. Aim higher. Second, waking up late doesn't mean before it's too late for the marriage to survive. Too late can mean irreparable injury to self-esteem, unrecoverable emotional distance, too many irretrievable hurtful words. Too late can also mean too late to model for your children what true intimacy looks like. Believe that children learn what they see, and if you want better for them, get better for yourself right now.

But This Wasn't My Idea

- When I was writing this book, a girlfriend said, "Don't give my husband something to use against me." If your husband brought this book home to you, you may be feeling hurt or offended. Try to keep an open mind.
- Show him—and remind yourself of—the passage that says a sexually disinterested woman is only half of the equation (see page 32).
- Consider the idea that he misses a connection that you once shared, not that he sees you as a sexual failure.

- Recognize that it takes courage for him to open the dialogue in a culture that tells him Real Men have women begging for more.
- Believe that you have the opportunity to be closer than ever, and now is the right time.

Take This Wonderful Opportunity

Chances are, you are reading this because you're out of the major denial stage. You may be extremely worried that something is wrong sexually or just a little concerned about the sexual blahs. I applaud you for tackling the subject wherever you're at on the spectrum. If the biggest issue is that things are just plain boring, good for you for jumping in early to get things rekindled. If, on the other hand, you haven't had sex for several months, even years, take credit for recognizing that it's never too late. It's natural to dread talking with your sexual partner about sexual difficulties. Be very proud of yourself for taking this step.

Affirmation
"Watch for big problems. They disguise big opportunities."
—H. Jackson Brown Jr., *Life's Little Instruction Book*

The Third Obstacle: Maternal Sacrifice

Aren't We Supposed to Give Up Our Lives?

> "Even with the profound changes that feminism and new economic times have brought, many mothers remain vulnerable to excessive guilt and self-blame. Mothers take their children's problems and unhappiness personally, even when the mothers themselves are desperately overworked . . ."
>
> —Harriet Lerner, *The Mother Dance: What Children Do to Your Life*

- A common source of sexual burnout is maternal burnout. Mothers who are exhausted from mothering are too tired for sex.
- Symptoms of excessive maternal sacrifice include frenzied parenting, a chronic sense of failing to live up to internal standards, and an inability to accept help.
- Your child almost certainly needs a less-stressed mother more than he needs another enriching activity.

Some of us had mothers like Sarah's; some of us had mothers like Sharon's:

> "I just want my kids to grow up having what I had as a child. I was so proud of my mom, and so lucky that she always put us first. I feel like I grew up on *Leave It to Beaver:* homemade cookies, picnics in the park, staged musicals in the basement. You name it, she did it. My kids deserve nothing less."
>
> —*Sarah, mother of two*

"I'm terrified that I'll turn out like my own mother. My earliest memories are of her sitting on the couch in front of a soap opera, half-blitzed, a cigarette about to burn a hole in the carpet. I'd kill myself if I ever thought I was even close to being that oblivious. What was she thinking?"
    —*Sharon, mother of one*

We judge ourselves as mothers, judge our own mothers, and judge our friends as they mother, often unaware that we are doing so. In an instant, we can describe a good mother, can tell you what good mothers do, say, and think. We know what good mothers feed their children, what good mothers allow kids to watch on television, what good mothers read to their children, and what good mothers do with their kids on Saturday afternoons. You can sum up our culture's requirement for "good" motherhood in a word: sacrifice.

Your internalized ideal mother is ridiculously perfect: She never raises her voice, always disciplines lovingly and calmly, remains two steps ahead of her child at all times, and soothes her toddler's scraped knee as ably as her teen's wounded heart. She gets her workout in by 5:30 A.M. because her kids hate the baby-sitting room at the gym. She doesn't beg her children to eat their salad. Instead, she serves crunchy snowman-shaped crudités that her children joyfully dip into low-fat ranch dressing. She uses her lunch hour to make sure that her preteen has the latest hot group's CD the first day it's in the store.

What's missing in the idealized mother image? (Besides reality!) Mom's needs. Mom's life. Mom's worries. Mom's relationships. Mom's time. Mom's body. Needless to say, mom's sexuality doesn't even register. Our culture tells us that good mothers are selfless, quick to sacrifice any and all of their own needs for the sake of their children.

The pressures on today's mother are higher than ever before in history. One of Freud's unrealistic legacies is the notion that mothers are entirely responsible for their children's emotional well-being. Or, as Harriet Lerner says, " . . . much of psychology remains a whodunit with the finger pointed in the mother's direction."[1] We obsess about empathic toilet training, use time-outs unless the experts tell us we're overdoing it, buy books on how to talk nicely to teenagers. The stakes are high, the payoff invisible, and mothers are constantly invited to step on the treadmill of maternal self-denial, leaving no energy for sex or anything else.

Excessive Sacrifice Leads to Sexual Depletion

Giving too much is a common source of maternal depletion, and tired moms are not interested in sex. Mothers tend to think of maternal fatigue as a simple day-to-day issue. We feel entitled to be tired when a sick child needs attention in the middle of the night or if we burn the midnight oil on a big work project. We understand the connection between a poor night's sleep and lack of sexual interest the following evening. But we often fail to recognize fatigue once it has become a way of life. You may not recognize that being too tired for sex isn't just an issue of being too tired at the end of an especially busy day.

   Women experience twice the rate of clinical depression as men, and I'm convinced that part of our increased vulnerability is our insistence that we can and must take care of everyone else's needs. Many mothers hold two contradictory ideas about nurturing. We endorse the idea that self-care is necessary for mothers while repeatedly failing to take care of ourselves. We may believe that it is enjoyable to give to others while at the same time blocking or ignoring the caretaking efforts of our friends and family.

[1] Harriet Lerner, "Enough Guilt for Now, Thank You," in *The Mother Dance* (New York: HarperCollins, 1999), p. 85.

Many of my patients make an unconscious contract with themselves: They'll nurture *until* they get depleted, and then, and only then, perhaps with the help of Prozac or Zoloft, they'll start to put their own needs on the agenda. The mothers that I see who are clinically depressed, beset by anxiety, or on the verge of divorce have almost always been ignoring the warning signals. Depletion doesn't announce itself like a train conductor, warning you of the last stop prior to burnout. One day you just arrive.

You know the warning signals: irritability, fatigue, tension, restless sleep, feeling overwhelmed, procrastination, angry outbursts. Symptoms of maternal depletion may be physical: headaches, neck stiffness, back pain, and frequent colds. But there is a very important symptom of maternal stress that you might have overlooked: *Sexual disinterest is a symptom of depletion.*

Exhausted mothers eventually run out of all resources, but typically the very first to go is sexual energy. Unless a woman really, really loves sex, she will quickly be too tired for sex. A mother who doesn't have time to get her hair cut doesn't have time for sex. A mother who constantly feels that she isn't measuring up to her own perfectionistic standard isn't going to feel good about herself in the bedroom or entitled to adult pleasures of any sort.

Here are statements by mothers who are simply too tired for sex.
1. "I rarely feel that I've done enough for my kids."
2. "When I take time for myself, I feel selfish."
3. "If my child has a problem at school, the first thing I think is that I have made a mistake."
4. "I often feel inadequate compared to other mothers."
5. "When I finally snap, I hear myself sounding like a martyr."
6. "When another mother describes a hobby or special

talent that her child participates in, I feel guilty, worried, envious, or anxious about whether I should have my child enrolled in that activity."

7. "I often feel that I am failing my parental duties by failing to provide enough enrichment for my children's lives."

Chances are you've got at least a touch of excessive sacrifice if you're a mom. Giving of yourself feels good, and I know as well as the next mom how intensely gratifying nurturing one's family can be. The problem is when we decide that if some is good, more is better. Maternal sacrifice is more like caffeine or alcohol than it is like kindness: Too much is simply too much. Unless you take care of yourself, you are unlikely to improve your libido.

What Kids Don't Need

Overzealous sacrificers typically believe that the only alternative to bullet-proof mothering is narcissistic, me-first self-indulgence. They think about their children's lives in stark black-or-white images: perfect or deprived, with nothing in between. It isn't so.

Saving some of you for yourself doesn't mean becoming a bad mother. It means embracing and really appreciating what the British pediatrician and psychoanalyst D. W. Winnicott called "good enough mothering." Not only is good enough mothering all that our children really need from us, it is all that we can provide.

Excessive sacrifice is not only doomed to fail, but ironically, it's not in your children's best interests either. Staying up all night hand stitching a gorgeous one-of-a-kind Halloween costume will leave you tired and cranky when your husband makes an overture, and you probably won't even enjoy the trick-or-treating. There are no exceptions to the rule that all mothers must make time for themselves.

One type of excessive sacrifice has been called "hyper-parenting."[2] This term refers to a mothering style that is rushed, busy, competitive, and frenzied. You run from Little League straight to ballet lesson, rarely linger over the family dinner table, and find that trying to "do nothing" as a family is more stressful than relaxing.

"Hyper-parenting" crept into American family life so gradually that we hardly noticed until it had us by the throat. As children, we probably played unattended in the backyard, with little parental concern that our futures might be harmed by unstructured games with the neighbor children. As mothers, we feel obligated to expose our children to the perfect array of planned educational and cultural experiences. We've been programmed to fear for our children's future, worried that anything we fail to provide them at just the right stage of development will ultimately harm their chances of getting into the right college, interfere with their self-esteem, or even keep them out of a good future career. This is a treadmill with no "off" switch. No wonder many mothers are too tired for sex!

Another hallmark of self-denying mothers is making themselves indispensable and being unable to delegate or let others—even husbands—help out. Indispensability is a seductive demon for mothers. It starts when our children are newborns and we experience the thrill of being the one best able to read our infant's cues, to soothe her in just the right way, to keep her feeling safe in the presence of strangers. We've all experienced the glow of being the one favored during times of sickness, the intoxication of having a toddler reach for our unique embrace. It simply feels great to be adored above all others.

[2]Alvin Rosenfeld and Nicole Wise, *Hyper-Parenting: Are You Hurting Your Child by Trying Too Hard?* (New York: St. Martin's Press, 2000).

Why do I call it a seductive demon? Because we can come to need that validation from our children. If we come to need the validation of our mothering, we can't let others in our child's "village" help out. If we come to believe that we and we alone are best able to meet our children's needs, guilt and anxiety quickly become the foundation of our mothering. We may also come to resent our husbands for not helping more, unaware of our own contribution to martyrdom: the subtle ways in which we prevent them from helping out more.

Indispensability may become a source of marital conflict, since mothers are far more likely than fathers to accept the mantle of perfect parenting. Busy fathers also may put romance on the back burner, but they are less inclined than mothers to allow sex to fade away. They may be more likely to ask for sex, and this may make matters worse, heightening the sense of sex as an obligation, a marital duty rather than a mutual experience. Along with being too tired for sex, you may be too annoyed with the burdens of family life to feel romantically inclined toward the partner you subconsciously pushed to the side.

What Kids Do Need

Let me assure you that kids do not need mothers who give too much. Good enough is truly good enough. Kids *do* thrive in a family where adult caretakers are deeply connected. If you want to do something for your children, pay attention to the threats to their parents' intimacy. Eventually, even great marriages sag under the weight of sexual distance.

In the year 2002, the average middle-class child is not going to suffer from one fewer piano lesson or bedtime story. Children are at far greater risk of growing up with parents who are cold and distant within their marriage or angry and resentful after divorce.

Unless you begin to take better care of yourself, I do not expect that your sex drive will go up, even if you follow every other piece of advice in this book! I'm being forceful here for a reason: I know how easy it is to believe that we are the exception, that there isn't enough time in the day, that self-care is selfish, that we'll get to it later, that someone's feelings will be hurt if we say no, or that creating limits on our availability would place an unfair burden on someone else.

What interferes with self-nurture? We know one easy answer: Women are socialized to be outwardly directed. From early on, the cultural script for women guides us to value connectedness. It teaches us to find pleasure in pleasing others, to feel a sense of accomplishment when we take care of others.

Please know that I'm not against caretaking! I love being a mother (most of the time), and I love being a doctor (most of the time). I am grateful that nurturing is compatible with femininity and grateful that I don't have to justify the limits at work that allow me to experience the pleasure of being deeply involved in my children's lives.

As a caretaker of women, however, I see all too often how one can have too much of a good thing. Day after day in my clinical work, I help exhausted women overcome psychological obstacles to self-care. In a later chapter, "Step Two: Safeguard Your Sexual Energy," I'll describe some strategies to help you cut back on excessive self-sacrifice. Here, I just want you to be honest with yourself about whether your mothering style is part of the problem.

We all know that we mothers are supposed to take care of ourselves, too. If you haven't been able to make this happen on your own so far, I hope that understanding that low libido is a symptom of chronic maternal fatigue will be the key that finally unlocks the door to self-nurture. Taking care of her own inner balance is every mother's obligation to herself.

Affirmation

" . . . as the overworked, exhausted parents of a generation of busy, overstimulated children, we can slow down the pace of daily life in our own homes. We can gently reshape lives that have become overstuffed and overly stressful. . . . We can protect and honor quiet, unscheduled time, and we can bequeath it to our sons and daughters."

—Katrina Kenison, *Mitten Strings for God: Reflections for Mothers in a Hurry*

The Fourth Obstacle: Disconnection

If Only Sex Were the Problem

> *"A couple's sex life is the most vulnerable part of the marriage. . . ."*
>
> —Judith Wallerstein, *Compassionate Marriage*

- Couples with intact emotional connectedness can have boring sex.
- Couples who are emotionally alienated are unlikely to have great sex or even mediocre sex.
- If anger and resentment are the basis of sexual disinterest, couples need to reconnect emotionally before seeking to reestablish sexual intimacy.

Having sex with someone you don't like all that much has no appeal. It's natural for women to lose interest in a sexual partner in the absence of loving feelings. But it doesn't necessarily follow that lack of sexual interest after children is a symptom of an underlying marital problem.

It's natural to experience anxiety about feeling either sexually or emotionally disconnected from one's partner. The secrets of lasting love in marriage can seem so elusive that some perfectly happily married moms are so vigilant they're almost paranoid—*too* worried about whether the sexual blahs are due to undetected emotional problems in the marriage. These readers may be reassured by knowing that the sexual issues are, indeed, sexual issues.

At the other extreme are women who are miserable in their marriages but terrified of admitting that emotional disconnection is the primary cause of sexual disconnection. If sexual distance is, in fact, a symptom of a troubled marriage, it's terribly important to address the relationship issues first. There are two reasons for this. First, restoring sexual passion requires trust and communication within a couple. You don't have to have a perfect marriage to revitalize your sex life, but you do need a fundamentally sound foundation upon which to rebuild. Second, attempting to put the cart before the horse won't work. Isolating sexual issues from the larger context of deep marital discontent actually may widen the emotional distance.

Finding the right place to start is so important that any responsible sex therapist looks first at the relationship.[1] This chapter can't substitute for a clinical evaluation, but if there is any doubt on your part whatsoever about the foundation of your marriage, please continue with this chapter. This book won't help you if the foundation of your marriage is crumbling due to addiction, flagrant hostility, abuse, hopeless miscommunication, or infidelity. In such marriages, low libido is a symptom of a larger problem, not the cause. That is why, for example, the first response to an affair shouldn't be sex therapy, because something is wrong with the infrastructure.

What's Wrong: Sexual Blahs as the Issue

The following checklist includes statements typical of mothers who are experiencing sexual issues in their marriages due to ordinary parenting stressors and poor habits. These statements suggest that monotony, boredom, depletion, and lack of opportunity are symptoms of benign neglect, not deep-seated problems. Agreement with many

[1] Equally important is ruling out physiological problems. See Step Ten.

of these statements suggests that the sexual "garden" needs attention—some freshening up, a bit of weeding, some fertilizer—not a
bulldozer.

Answer "true" or "false" for each statement.

1. "Given the choice between a quickie and getting fifteen more minutes of sleep, I'll choose sleep."
2. "My nightclothes could pass inspection at the Vatican."
3. "My mind wanders when making love, sometimes to things as mundane as the next day's carpool schedule or what's happening at the office."
4. "The second I climax, I wish my husband would hurry up and climax too so that I could get to sleep."
5. "I would describe our lovemaking as 'efficient.'"
6. "When we make love, chances are that it will be just like the last ten times we made love."
7. "I can't remember the last time one of us tried to introduce something new to our lovemaking."
8. "If you tallied up the time per week that we spend really kissing passionately, it would add up to less than the time we spend emptying the garbage."
9. "I keep a mental calendar in my head of when we last made love, to help me decide whether it's okay to say no if I'm not in the mood."
10. "Sometimes I just feel like kissing and caressing, but I don't even do that because if I already know I'm not in the mood for sex, I don't want my husband to get annoyed or frustrated."
11. "Although I don't initiate sex as often as my husband does, once we get going, I usually enjoy it."

12. "On vacation, my sexual energy comes back."
13. "I miss sex if we haven't had time to make love lately."
14. "If my husband and I had a weekend alone with no children, we'd both be looking forward to the sexual opportunities."

Evaluating Your Answers

The first eight statements are classic symptoms of the sexual monotony common among busy parents. For tired mothers, sex is largely conducted on autopilot. No one sets out to make sex boring; you get there one tiny step at a time. The good news is that you can get your sexual groove back by making better choices and small but meaningful changes.

Statements 9 and 10 are yellow warning signs of potential trouble ahead. They may indicate that sex is becoming an obligation, and that guilt, pressure, or a sense of duty has entered the sexual relationship. Occasionally saying yes when you really don't feel like it is just one of the compromises people who love each other make. In a sense, it's not unlike deciding how to spend time in other ways: someone gets to pick the movie, the restaurant, or the vacation destination when there isn't consensus. But duty sex can quickly become a heavy burden that backfires. Mothers who frequently feel coerced or guilt-tripped into having sex become progressively less interested. It is important to take action to avoid the downward spiral in which sex as a duty quickly annihilates sex as a pleasure.

Figuring out where you fall on the spectrum of duty sex helps steer you in the right direction. Some women never initiate sex, but enjoy it once it gets going (statement 11). This is not pathological, but rather is like not thinking about dessert yet still enjoying it once it's in front of you. It's important to know that one common sexual difference among husbands and wives is that a significant number of women are primarily reactive to sexual overtures. The key is that sex is enjoyable once underway. It isn't an imposition, it's just not something you initiate.

However, you don't have to settle for always being the invitee. Sexual anticipation is part of the pleasure, and it would be great to enjoy the anticipation as well as the lovemaking itself. The steps described in this book will help you take charge of your own sexuality. You'll remember how great it is to want sex, and I guarantee that your husband will be delighted to share the responsibility for initiating sex.

At the other end of the spectrum are women for whom sex is *only* an unwanted obligation. This is often due to a significant marital problem (more about this later). However, if you once enjoyed lovemaking with your partner but now hate it, and you feel that your relationship is emotionally intimate, it is absolutely essential to have a physical evaluation to rule out a medical cause (see Step 10). In the absence of physical or marital problems, sex can become a duty simply because it's boring. If you find that using the steps in this book doesn't alleviate the burden of lovemaking, you might benefit from professional help.

Prognosis: Excellent

The last three statements indicate a good prognosis. Lovemaking has remained enjoyable, and sexual energy is a renewable resource. This is an excellent time to intervene, because you already know that sex is great when it's great. The challenge for you is to make great sex the rule rather than the exception.

Why Would I Want to Have Sex with Him?

Many so-so marriages limp along, tolerable if not fabulous, until children are born. Raising children is often the single biggest challenge couples face together, and weakness in a marriage is magnified during this period. If sexual and relationship problems first appear after children arrive, many couples will mistakenly attribute sexual dissatisfaction to fatigue or the physical changes of childbirth. The following section will help you take a look at whether your marriage has deeper relationship problems outside the bedroom.

Be honest.

I know it's frightening to acknowledge being in an unhappy marriage, but sex therapy and three months alone together on a deserted island won't help your sex life if you don't address underlying relationship issues.

Sexual problems are almost certainly a symptom rather than a cause of marital unhappiness if you've begun to fantasize or contemplate the end of your marriage. Also, scorn, disgust, contempt, ridicule, loneliness, and fear are major signs of toxicity in a marriage. It's only natural to lack sexual interest in a spouse one doesn't like or one who disrespects you. Other worrisome changes are sexual untruths, sexual sacrifice, and anger or victimization in response to a partner's interest or disinterest in sex.

Answer "true" or "false" for each statement.

1. "It's more peaceful at home when I say yes to sex more often than I'd like to, because he's really cranky or withholding if we haven't had sex lately. The truth is, I've had plenty of sex when I didn't want to just to get him to be nicer to me."

2. "I dread having my husband initiate sex."
3. "If I'm having difficulty reaching climax, I'll pretend to have an orgasm."
4. "My husband is often scornful of how I spend money, use my time, and/or keep house."
5. "I sometimes fantasize about being widowed or divorced."
6. "When we argue, I often feel attacked and defensive. Our arguments quickly escalate, and one or both of us bring up something that's been simmering for a while."
7. "When he doesn't like something I've done, he'll tease me or embarrass me in front of friends or family by telling the story of what I did or didn't do."
8. "My husband doesn't do his fair share around the house. I'm what's meant by the term married single mom: I have all the drawbacks of divorce without any of the benefits."
9. "I feel lonely within my marriage."
10. "I don't respect my husband the way I did when we were first married. If it weren't for the children, I don't think we'd still be together."

If you agree with more than one or two of the above statements, you may feel panicky right now. Or you may feel sad or oddly relieved to have your worst fear confirmed. It's a matter of personal difference in how you handle uncomfortable news. Some people don't want the biopsy results; others just want to know the diagnosis as quickly as possible. The "diagnosis" of what is wrong is just like a biopsy result: The label doesn't change reality, it simply helps you figure out how to develop solutions.

This book will primarily address issues of depletion, boredom, and mismatched libidos. If you see from your self-diagnosis that the primary issue in your sexual relationship is significant marital unhappiness, I encourage you to develop a plan of action in addition to using this book. My favorite self-help book on marriage rebuilding is John Mordechai Gottman and Nan Silver's book, *The Seven Principles for Making Marriage Work*. I also often recommend Phillip C. McGraw's *Relationship Rescue*. Consider couples counseling, as described in Step Ten. Get moving. The sexual health of the marriage is unlikely to improve in the absence of a solid emotional foundation. The two are not mutually exclusive, and there are ideas and suggestions in this book that foster sexual communication at the same time that you are rebuilding the basics of emotional trust and connection.

For the remainder of the readers, we're ready to move on to the Ten Steps to Nurturing Passion.

Affirmation

"For although in sexual love we may strive to continue with our body the connections we have made with our heart and our mind, there are times when the leap from love to ecstasy fails. There are times—there are plenty of times—when what we will have to settle for are imperfect connections."
—Judith Viorst, *Necessary Losses*

The
Prescription

Phase One
ESTABLISH a FOUNDATION of VALUES

The first three steps toward reclaiming passion all involve examining and reworking your core beliefs about mothering and sexuality.

Before the kids arrived, sexual privacy was a no-brainer. As long as you didn't have sex while you had dinner guests, maintaining sexual boundaries was not an issue. These days, the biggest sexual challenge of all may be logistical.

And, almost certainly, in the early days, you had time for yourself. It didn't seem selfish to make sure that you had sexual energy before energy became so scarce. Even the Marine Corps doesn't expect from its forces what children ask of their moms. Chances are you never had sex with such a demanding taskmaster running your life.

Values are beliefs about what should happen. Values come with labels: good or bad, right or wrong. Values also exist in a hierarchy: What's most important? What should be sacrificed for the greater good?

Values about sexuality (e.g., sex is an important and enjoyable aspect of an intimate relationship) commonly conflict with values about mothering (e.g., the highest priority is meeting the perceived needs of the children). I'm going to challenge you to establish a foundation of values that will allow you to integrate great sex with great mothering.

Another value I'm going to ask you to examine is the core belief you have about what "nice girls" do. If there is a silver lining to the negative impact of children on sexuality, it is that you can, once and for all, decide to turn off the internal censor that expresses Puritanical disapproval at anything that isn't plain vanilla. When you first discover plain vanilla, it's fantastic. After a while, it gets old. After kids, it gets very old.

Now is the time to value your sexual creativity.

The first three steps build a foundation of values for great sex for moms.

Before you can have great sex again, you must feel entitled to it.

You must believe that you are permitted to stay sexual as a responsible parent.

You must believe that preserving your sexual energy is necessary.

And you must believe that you are the best judge of what is sexually appropriate within your own bedroom.

Step One: Honor Parental Sexuality as a Family Value

"Is a parent's lot all sacrifice until the geriatrician becomes our personal physician?"

—Alvin Rosenfeld, M.D., and Nicole Wise, *Hyper-Parenting: Are You Hurting Your Child by Trying Too Hard?*

- A good parental sex life is important for a strong family.
- What you model at home is your best opportunity to counteract the negative cultural messages about sexuality that your children get in every other arena of their lives.
- You have the right to sexual privacy and sexual boundaries within your home.

The mythical ideal of infinite maternal devotion and selflessness is incompatible with having a life, sexual or otherwise. It's too exhausting trying to be the heroic Perfect Mother. Just as me-only time is an important part of being the best mother you can be, couple-only time, including time for relaxed sexual intimacy, is an important part of being the strongest family you can be.

Why is good sex so important to a family? Can something invisible to children be so good for them? You bet. Kids have a tremendous stake in their parents' intimacy. Intimate parents are more resilient, more affectionate, more peace-minded and forgiving. Intimate couples function better as a team, and that's good for kids.

Besides, it isn't so invisible. At some level, today's kids register that families are vulnerable. Every child knows someone with divorced parents. Seeing genuine affection expressed at home is reassuring for them.

Unfortunately, the Goodmans know only too well how hard it is to find couple time:

> Judy and Steve, parents of ten- and thirteen-year-old children, stay up until the children fall asleep. This was fine when the kids were asleep by 8:00 P.M. These days, though bedtime is officially 9:00 P.M. on school nights, enforcement is lax. One child will wander in complaining she can't sleep, or the other will suddenly remember he's hungry or forgot to brush his teeth. By the time both kids are asleep, Judy is usually too tired for lovemaking. Weekend and vacations are open season, with parents all too often falling asleep before the kids. They worry about the kids walking in, and it always seems too awkward to make love while they're awake. Steve wishes Judy would find the energy more often; Judy wishes Steve would get off her case. It's not her fault the kids won't give them any time alone. Both assume that they are helpless to change what the kids do.

Question Your Assumptions About Sexuality

Parents often consciously or unconsciously assume that once the kids are grown, things will be back to normal sexually. They believe marriage can readily withstand years of sexual mediocrity. Sex is sacrificed to the perceived needs of the children, much like we might put off buying a new car in order to save for their college funds.

The problem is that sex isn't a commodity that collects interest in the bank. Postponing adult sexuality is a sacrifice that actually isn't in your children's best interests, and, paradoxically, may harm them. Divorce presents an ever-present risk to American families, yet we continue to insist that the couple needs of parents belong on the back burner.

Often, until this is brought out into the open, the couple has not been aware of the unwritten contract to sacrifice this important aspect of the relationship. Like other assumptions of how any marriage operates, one partner may have decided this for the couple, leaving the other feeling excluded and disgruntled by what feels like a unilateral decree.

Be sure that you have really listened to what your spouse is saying about your sexual relationship and that he is listening to your concerns. Is it possible that one member of the couple has chosen to ignore the other partner's sexual unhappiness? Many spouses wind up stunned to discover that the other one has such serious concerns about the relationship. More often than we might want to admit, these unresolved issues are precursors to divorce.

Even if divorce is not a potential issue, ignoring the lack of sexual passion is not any more in your children's best interests than is ignoring an absence of love. Parents justify deferring sexual intimacy because they believe that children will be damaged if they so much as suspect that their parents are having sex. Parents often accept this as fact, just part of what it means to be good caretakers.

This is a legacy from Freudian psychology, highly specific to middle-class America. Freud believed that witnessing the "primal scene" (seeing your parents make love) would cause neurosis, in part because he believed the central psychological developmental issue in a child's life was resolving the impossible wish to marry one's opposite-sex parent. The theory that a single emotional upset would damage a child's psyche for life is at the root of frantic, perfectionistic, unattainable parenting. Think about it for a moment. Most people on the planet, most people in history, live or lived with whole families in one room. Laura Ingalls Wilder never mentioned hearing her sister be conceived, but you and I both know that the Little House on the Prairie was little.

I am not encouraging you to disregard appropriate sexual boundaries. However, I am disputing Freud's idea that the risk of a child accidentally overhearing or seeing lovemaking is so potentially psychologically damaging that the only acceptable alternative for good parents is to more or less give up sex.

Instead, use reasonable precautions but understand that as occasional parental sins go, the risk to your kids' well-being of accidental exposure to parental intimacy is not even on a par with forgetting to fasten their seatbelts.

What Do You Want Your Kids to Learn About Sexuality?

It is absurd to try to provide our children with a perfect environment. Ironically, while we zealously "protect" our children from seeing their parents as sexual beings, we relinquish our only opportunity to teach them our family's values about sexuality. We miss the opportunity to teach our children that love and physical intimacy go together, and this important message is too often exactly opposite what they see in the media.

Our kids are relentlessly exposed to sexual images, from perfect Barbie breasts to seductively gyrating teens on MTV to prime-time sitcoms that all too often tell our kids that sex is about anything but love, commitment, or respect. By scrupulously avoiding any gesture of affection beyond the most lifeless peck in front of the children, we reinforce the message that sex is not part of marriage. We tacitly concur that sex is only for the beautiful, the violent, the young, or that it is a forbidden pleasure—not for real moms and dads who love each other.

I'm not in favor of sexual indiscretion in the home. I don't think you should walk around naked, announce at breakfast that you had great sex last night, or put a sign on the bedroom door that says LOVEMAKING IN PROGRESS, DO NOT DISTURB. Simply demonstrate appropriate physical affection (such as a real kiss or hug) in front of your children.

It won't encourage premature sexual behavior. If only helping kids make good sexual choices were so simple! We can't just tell our kids to ignore what the rest of the culture says about sex having nothing to do with love, let alone marriage. We shouldn't pretend that if they don't know that we have sex, they won't ever do it.

We can model how love is connected to physical affection in our own lives. Never keeping a drop of alcohol in the house won't keep kids from experimenting with it elsewhere, and we can't expect our children to abstain if they see us drunk. It is quite possible, however, that seeing parents drink moderately and responsibly models exactly what we hope our kids will choose. So it is with appropriate marital affection.

Assumptions About Children's Needs

Parents assume that the needs and wishes of the children always trump their own. Certainly, one doesn't let a baby cry because his parents are making love or lock a preschooler out of the bedroom when she wakes up with an earache.

The all-consuming needs of very young children eventually diminish, but most parents don't consciously get out of the habit of 24/7 on-call status as their children age. This is what your grandmother would call spoiling them—acquiescing to a child's wish (here, an always available Mom) when a loving limit is a better gift. Here, the loving limit, the "no" that really is good for them, is private couple time.

In the absence of limits, children are always potential intruders in their parents' sex lives. Without privacy, parents have neither time nor space to foster intimacy. It is up to the parents to implement sexual boundaries—and here's how to do it.

Construct a Mission Statement

Children do learn what they live, and you and your spouse may wish to sit down and identify the family values about sexuality and/or parental needs that you want your children to learn. Creating a mission statement establishes a framework that helps guide your response to the inevitable challenges to parental boundaries. It also serves to remind us how we ourselves wish to respond to the endless opportunities to gently shape our children's understanding of the world. Mission statements are as ancient as the Ten Commandments and as modern as a dot-com industry's Powerpoint vision statement. It's a useful way to elucidate what you decide matters.

Once you've constructed your mission statement (and if you can't get your husband to participate, at least try to get him to sign off on yours), become mindful of the opportunity to discuss your values in parenting moments large and small. If your son demands a PB&J right this second because he doesn't want to miss the next *Rugrats* episode, take the opportunity to remind him that you take care of him but aren't willing to be his servant. When the tabloid at the grocery store announces that a heartthrob actor is leaving his wife because he's actually gay, mention to your teen that you think celebrities should be entitled to sexual privacy. If your ten-year-old claims that the baby-sitter is boring and you and Daddy never stay home, talk about how important alone time is for couples.

As an example to get you started, here are some messages for kids:

Parents have lives, too.

A closed door means do not enter without permission.

Being a mom is a joy, not a burden.

Just because I'm in the house doesn't mean I'm at your beck and call.

A mom kisses her kids one way, and the adult she loves romantically another way.

As you get older, it is appropriate to put yourself to bed, although I will remind you to brush your teeth until you go to college.

Parts of my life are none of my children's business.

There is enough of me for you and for me.

Nonsexual boundaries for parents are established when:

- Kids are fed first and parents enjoy a leisurely breakfast or dinner by themselves;
- Children are discouraged from interrupting phone calls;
- Mom takes a fifteen-minute break every day;
- Dad takes the kids to the baby-sitting room at the health club for his workout, even if they complain that it's boring;
- Children learn to sit quietly during religious services.

Sexual Privacy and Boundaries

Sexual privacy is the concealment and separation of adult intimacy from the world of children. A locked door and a night away are examples of parental sexual privacy. In contrast, I use the term "sexual boundary" psychologically. A sexual boundary is an imaginary circumference that demarcates this particular aspect of the non-mommy self. Imagine it as a protective fence surrounding a field where you can play safely.

> Become aware of every locked room in the house. Is there a guest room in the basement that locks? A bathroom?
>
> Any place that you can have sexual privacy is acceptable, and having more than one is ideal, especially if you allow kids to join the parents' bed freely (as some parents do secretly, others by choice as a policy). If you do have an open-bed policy, you must have some welcoming sexual space with a locked door elsewhere.

It is important for moms to create both sexual privacy and sexual boundaries. Locks alone are not enough. Believing that your sexual self is essential to family well-being is a sexual boundary. The decision to miss a child's basketball game in order to take twenty-four hours downtown with your husband is a sexual boundary. The fence that allows you to play safely inside also keeps out excessive self-sacrifice. In order to foster your sexual being, you will need a boundary that allows you "off-duty" mom time.

First, Get Some Good Locks

As children begin to wander the house independently, you must have a bedroom door lock and use it. The earlier that kids learn to respect the privacy of the parental bedroom, the better, but it's never too late to get a locksmith out to the house. The lock gives you thirty seconds to compose yourself before opening the door to your child. Perhaps more important, privacy is a prerequisite of a good sexual boundary.

You won't be able to relax and immerse yourself in lovemaking if you're worried that tonight just might be the first time in a year that little Joey wakes up and walks in unannounced.

To reclaim your privacy, you need to demonstrate that you honor the kids' privacy, too. Sooner or later, most mothers are tempted to intrude on a child's privacy. Reading a teenager's journal is easily rationalized as trying to be sure that they aren't getting into serious trouble. Walking in on the bath of a seven-year-old who just announced she wants privacy is awfully convenient when you need the box of Band-Aids from the medicine cabinet. Don't do it. Create an environment in which privacy is a family value.

When a child asks for privacy, whether it's a toddler wanting to go potty by herself or a teen declaring his room off limits, take the opportunity to discuss your own need for privacy. Respond with "I think that's a great idea, and I would like all of us to try to be more respectful of closed doors. Let's have a policy of knocking and then waiting to be invited to come in."

Ten Items That Passionate Parents Should Have and Use
The following help parents establish sexual boundaries and privacy:

1. a lock on the bedroom door;
2. a white-noise machine, loud humidifier, fan, radio, or boom-box that can be moved close to the door;
3. an off switch on the bedroom phone;
4. private space with a lock for storing anything you'd like your kids not to see (a file cabinet, tool box, or desk drawer works);
5. a non-mom, non-dad set of sleeping wear;

6. one nice set of underclothes for each;
7. a reliable baby-sitter;
8. a jar for loose change, designated to fund an occasional romantic adults-only evening or weekend at a hotel;
9. massage oil;
10. effective birth control any time you aren't intending to get pregnant.

Age-appropriate Solutions

Obtaining sexual privacy is a challenging task for parents of infants and toddlers. When they want us, they generally *need* us, and it is appropriate to defer your sexual moment to soothe a screaming infant or a scared toddler. Fortunately, the fact that they can't get out of the crib gives you potential sexual privacy (depending on whether you have ambulatory older children), but you have to plan for it. Parents of small children usually must think out sex in advance. One specific strategy is to plan time for lovemaking when the baby naps. Parents of very small children can also establish sexual boundaries by deciding to take time for sexuality, such as keeping the baby-sitter an extra hour while you kiss and snuggle in the car, dropping the baby at Grandma's while you run home and make love, or trading an overnight with friends who have a child.

As children grow up, we tend to miss the fact that sometimes when they want us, they *don't need* us. Judy and Steve hadn't intended to end up with their kids imposing on their couple time—it just seemed to end up that way. They decided to insist on adult time by implementing an "off-duty" rule, a designated time after which only dire emergencies were permitted interruptions. After some early adjustment issues, the children adapted once the rules were consistently enforced. In the new routine, at 8:30 P.M., everyone moves into gear to begin settling down. The parents help their children anticipate their needs: Are they hungry? Did they brush their teeth? Do they have something to read? The kids are not expected to be asleep by 9:00 P.M., but the parents established the clear expectation that kids stay in their rooms thereafter, engaging in quiet activities until they fall asleep.

The parents go "off duty" at 9:00 P.M. They don't make love until they know the kids are asleep, usually close to ten on school nights, but Judy and Steve found that having time to themselves every weeknight helped them reconnect emotionally and let each of them unwind before considering whether they wanted to make love. The rules remained relaxed on weekends and vacations, but they were pleased to find that they were both more likely to be in the mood when the opportunity arose.

Judy isn't comfortable making love while any child is awake, and she feels certain that she'd never be able to relax enough to enjoy it, even with a lock. She isn't really that worried about whether it would hurt them, but she cringes with mortification at the thought of being discovered having sex by anyone, let alone her own kids. If she were open to considering making love behind a locked door before she is certain everyone is asleep, she might find that a white-noise machine (or a radio or humidifier) placed near the door gave her the sexual boundary she needs to feel comfortable.

Some couples find sexual privacy by making a deliberate effort to be home alone and to pounce on the opportunity. For some, this means meeting at home on a school day during lunch, a solution that is practical only for parents with flexible work schedules. Others schedule overnight camp for the kids over the summer and enjoy an annual second honeymoon. One mom described her battle plan: She has found it much easier to make plans for one child when a sibling has been invited for a weekend sleepover. She will call the mom of her other child's best friend and tell a little white lie, such as "Heather was invited for a sleepover tonight. I was going to have her baby-sit Keith while we went to see a movie. If I took your boys next Saturday night, would Keith be able to visit Mark tonight?" Similarly, she might ask her mother to take them both to see the newest kid movie so that she and her husband could have a "date." Others occasionally set the alarm clock for sex at 4:00 A.M., especially on a morning when the kids are likely to let you sleep late.

What If the Worst Happens?

The single most distracting thought that goes through a mother's head during lovemaking generally starts with "What if the kids . . ." (wake up, walk in, hear us, etc.). It is understandable to be concerned about exposing the children inappropriately. But you may have given this possibility more significance than it deserves. Prevention—good locks—is the best strategy. If that fails, let's walk through the worst-case scenario.

Your child walks in on you and your husband making love. A younger child is unlikely to understand what is happening and may be frightened by the sound or sight of lovemaking. Address your child's fear. You will need to explain that moms and dads have a way of touching each other in private that adults really like but that may seem scary to kids. Matter-of-factly reassure him that no one was hurting and that this way of touching one another is something only grown-ups do.

A primary school–aged child may be quite curious without being frightened. Depending on your comfort level, you may wish to cut the why-is-the-sky-blue question-and-answer session to a minimum. Stick to the principle of saying only what is necessary to move to the next subject without shaming or inadvertently stirring up even more interest. Try "I can see that you're really curious about what you were hearing, but as you can see, we're fine. Sometimes adults do stuff kids don't understand yet." Then change the subject.

An older child may understand exactly what is happening and may be repulsed or embarrassed, not unlike what we feel if we imagine the thought of our own parents having sex. Your older child uses the same defense mechanisms you do when picturing parental sex: denial and suppression. He clicks the off switch and will be happy for you to let him retain plausible deniability. If an older child bursts in and the truth cannot be denied, don't fabricate or get defensive. Get dressed and talk about what happened. Acknowledge that this is awkward for all of you. Try "I guess you know what was happening just now. I know this is embarrassing for all of us, and that we'd all like to keep Mom and Dad's love life private." Discuss the steps to take next time to ensure privacy, without blaming your child or yourself. I can promise you a very brief conversation.

It's Good for Everyone

The rest of this book assumes that you will give yourself the gift of sex. This is also a gift to your children, whether they know it. Couple time is not selfish indulgence by parents—it's part of a healthy family. Just because it sounds so great to the mother doesn't mean it's bad for the kids!

Affirmation
"A wise man will make more opportunities than he finds."
　　　—Francis Bacon

Step Two: Safeguard Your Sexual Energy

> "When do we start to feel guilty about pursuing pleasure and play? At what stage of development do we adopt the belief that our larger purpose is to serve everyone else's needs?"
>
> —Alice Domar and Henry Dreher, *Self-Nurture*

- Stress reduction is libido enhancement. Excessive service to others is a major sexual drain for mothers.
- You can boost your sex drive and care for yourself at the same time.
- Perfectionism is a sexual antagonist that can be overcome by changing how you think about mothering.

Stress and fatigue are the natural enemies of a mother's sex drive. Honoring your own need for renewal is an important value that establishes the foundation for great sex.

There is no shortage of advice on how to reduce maternal stress. Whether you connect to women's media via the Internet, watch Oprah, or subscribe to *Redbook*, chances are you've encountered a list of "stress-busters." Advice on reducing stress is a lot like advice on weight loss: You can fancy it up, but it still basically boils down to a simple mathematical formula. To reduce weight, we have to eat fewer calories or burn more. Period. To reduce stress, we have to consume less of our own energy or find new sources. Period. Do less for others or self-nurture more. Drain the batteries less or recharge them more often.

Self-care is a lifestyle choice. Self-care is the natural outgrowth of believing that you matter, too. It is not a secret or a myth, and there are no shortcuts.

Visualize Your "Caretaker Profile"

Of all the aspects of motherhood that interfere with sexual desire, for many women, caretaking of others is the biggest offender. Many mothers feel that the *only* place no one needs anything is bed. The *only* just-me time is at the end of the day. A sexual overture in that place, at that time, is often experienced by burned-out mothers as a call to service, the last on a list of should-do's that made up her day. Step Two toward reestablishing sexual intimacy as a pleasure rather than a duty is to clear some time and space other than the bedroom for me-only time, and put sexual self-nurture back in your life. I'll show you how.

It's easy for mothers to ignore how unmanageable the duty roster has become. Visualization is a great way to become aware of a truth you've been avoiding. Draw a circle that represents you in your wakeful hours. Using a pie-graph model, honestly indicate how much of your circle is devoted to caretaking. These duties may be pleasurable, such as watching soccer practice, or they may be loathsome, such as cleaning the refrigerator or changing cat litter, but include all the things in a typical week that you should or must do. Use the other part of the pie to indicate how much of your circle is non-obligatory. These activities include anything that doesn't serve or benefit anyone else but you.

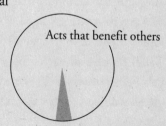

Acts that benefit others

Things I do for myself

How much of your circle is devoted to service to others? How much is just for you? Look at the kinds of things commonly found on a mother's duty roster: prepare meals; organize backpacks; carpool; do laundry and dishes; fill out school, camp, and club forms; help with homework; volunteer at school; care for pets; arrange doctor and dentist appointments.

If you work outside the home, how much of your professional life is spent serving others? Do clients, customers, employees, coworkers, or bosses compete for your caretaking? What is the balance at the office between what you get and what you give?

Sometimes it's easy to get where you're going as long as you decide where you want to be. Use the pie graph visualization to set a destination. Commit to widening the portion of unobligated activities. Start with a sliver if that's the best you can do for now. Go back every few weeks and revisit your pie chart and see if you can't widen the sliver a tiny bit more. You will know which me-only activities to add—what brings you pleasure, what's affordable, what's feasible. Decide to go there. It's not easy, but it can be done.

Here are some examples of things that you can do to widen the me-only portion of your life: buy yourself flowers, browse a bookstore, meet a friend for coffee (one who doesn't need any help), get a free makeover at a department store, shut the door at work and read a magazine for ten minutes, schedule a time-off break of fifteen minutes at home and insist that the kids occupy themselves then.

I can hear you saying "I would if I had time." Okay, so how much time *do* you have to spare? Ideally, I'd like to see every mother take Sarah Ban Breathnach's suggestion of scheduling two hours for herself before she puts in the rest of the week's activities.[1] Practically, many women simply can't or won't do so.

---

[1] Sarah Ban Breathnach, *Simple Abundance* (New York: Warner Books, 1995).

As a first step, I will settle for whatever time you decide that you can spare. Be specific: How many minutes per day or week can you redirect toward self-care? If it's two hours a week, consider activities that "feed" you: creativity (an arts class), intellectual stimulation (a lecture or a book), relaxation (gardening or doing yoga). If exercise is a pleasure and not a duty, an aerobic workout is a proven libido booster. If you can find only fifteen minutes a week, make the most of it. A luxurious bath with aromatherapy salts, coffee, and the newspaper, or a brief rest in the backyard soaking up the sun's warmth are renewing but cost little time. If you can spare only a minute a day, try the following: Close your eyes, breathe deeply, and make your eyelids as heavy as possible, then visualize a wave of muscle relaxation flowing down from the top of your head, into your neck and shoulders, and down your torso and legs, into the tips of your toes. Try to repeat this minute later in the day.

The actual clock time that you spend on yourself is very important in regaining balance. Equally important is the discipline and intentionality of doing something for yourself, however small. Deciding to add even a small moment of self-soothing on a regular basis is in and of itself self-care. Taking a relaxing minute each day is a way of becoming mindful of your own needs, of remaining aware that you matter, too. You will be surprised at how easy it is to find more than a minute a day once you see the benefits of self-nurture each and every day. Over time, self-care creates energy that can be channeled into lovemaking.

Self-nurture Can Be Sexy, Too

For mothers, relaxation as a means of getting in the mood cannot be overemphasized. Destressing to reduce baseline fatigue as just described is part of a sexual overhaul. Take it up a notch and schedule specific sensuality recharging days.

A libido-boosting day consists of intense relaxation in combination with activities that get sexual thoughts flowing and/or honor your body as a source of physical pleasure. Many women find that they just don't have the libido on-off switch that their husbands possess, making a slow buildup essential.

If you've hit a brick wall trying to get your husband to take more responsibility caring for the kids, try suggesting that he gets the kids next Saturday while you rev your sexual engine. Be playful and avoid taking the discussion up a notch about what's unfair in the division of labor. Explain that you're experimenting with different approaches so that you don't feel pressured to perform sexually at the end of the day.

At first, it may take discipline and structure to incorporate active libido boosting into your schedule. Think of this as being like working out: It never seems like you have the time until you're hooked. Give this approach a try and stay open to the idea that the benefits only become clear with repetition.

Sexy Self-nurturing Activities

- Go to an afternoon romantic and sexy R-rated movie by yourself or with a girlfriend.
- Shop for a beautiful camisole and wear it home.
- Go to the library and read *Cosmo,* especially about things you'd never do in a million years.
- Get a massage (some health food stores now offer quickies for very reasonable prices; get as much time as you can afford).
- Read a sexy or romantic novel anywhere but at home.
- Sit in a coffee shop and write down the details of the time you conceived your child. Be explicit!
- Watch couples kissing in public.

- Go to a bookstore in a neighborhood where no one knows you and look through books on sexuality.
- Buy candles to light that night. Spend at least a half an hour enjoying the variety of smells. Test the hypothesis that food scents (pumpkin, vanilla, clove) are libido building.
- Work out shortly before you head home. (Exercise increases pelvic blood flow and releases hormones that stimulate sex drive and make climax easier for some women.)
- Write erotic haiku (three-line poems that follow a five-/seven-/five-syllable pattern) in a café.
- Avoid alcohol, which actually decreases sex drive, makes you sleepier, counteracts all that you've done to lift your energy, and makes climax less likely.

When You Get Home That Night

- Inform the kids that Dad is in charge of bedtime tonight. Resist the nonverbal invitations to help out, whether from him or the kids.
- Get involved in something that signals that you are not available or put up a DO NOT DISTURB MOMMY sign. Lock yourself in the bathroom, take a bubble bath, and read that sexy novel some more. Tell your husband to give you a knock that signals the coast is clear.
- Take an early-evening nap (the single most effective way to boost your sexual energy later that night).
- If it's warm enough, sit in the backyard. Remember a scene from the movie you saw earlier, or the book you read, and practice fantasizing about the best scenes.

Take Stress and Duty Off Your List

The strategies mentioned so far are ways to nurture yourself. The flip side of self-care is less self-depletion. In addition to self-nurture, creating a foundation of sexuality-friendly values will probably mean that you have to eliminate some sources of maternal drain. Seeing your duty profile in black and white may be all that it takes to get back in balance. Still, most moms have an ongoing struggle with identifying which duties can be delegated, which can be hired out, which can be eliminated altogether, and which can be done less thoroughly.

It may seem that sex was better in the beginning of the relationship because it was fresh, but don't underestimate the fact that you had oodles of time to yourself in those days. *You* were fresh when you set out to make love. If you really are going to choose to make your own needs matter, chances are that you will need to let go of some of the tasks that drain your sexual energy.

One dramatic change is to stop "service hemorrhages." Is there a coworker, a relative, or a friend who is sucking you dry? This is the person whose phone number you hate to see on Caller ID, the one you hope doesn't ask you to lunch, the friend who lives from crisis to crisis. We are so socialized to nurture and support others that we often confuse caretaking with rescuing; we ignore the sinking feeling that signals a lack of reciprocity. Or we feel guilty. What kind of woman would refuse to help someone in crisis (never mind that it's the seventh one this month)?

To stop energy-depleting caretaking, pay more attention to your gut. If you're in a relationship that hasn't ever and won't ever be mutual, it isn't good for you and, truly, it isn't good for your friend, relative, or coworker, either. Stop responding to the invitation to pretend to solve her problems, to play "yes but" (in which you offer suggestions that she promptly rejects), or to serve as her dumping ground. Respond to her unloading with an action *she* must take. Say, "Gee, that sounds awful. What are you going to do about it?" Or "Maybe a therapist could help you deal with all the feelings you have about your husband's drinking/your abusive boss/your mother's criticisms/your ex/etc." Or "I think you should talk to someone in personnel about this situation." Limit your availability, honestly and kindly: "Hi, Nancy. Listen, I have only five minutes. What is on your mind?" Serving as someone's on-call stress-release valve is not part of a value system that honors and safeguards sexual energy.

Mothers are often called to Herculean tasks on behalf of the organizations that serve their children. Just say no. Do not run the Girl Scout cookie sale if you want to enjoy sex in the next three months. I promise, the cookies will get sold. There is always a mom who thrives on martyrdom, and you can't change her. Never, never, never say yes because you feel sorry for another mom who always says yes. If you take the school carnival off her hands, she's going to say yes to something else.

Here are three ways to say no without feeling guilty. First, say no to the energy-draining activity at the same time that you say yes to something manageable. "I won't be able to chair the pancake breakfast, but put me down for working a shift that day." Or say a soft but firm no: "I don't think I can take that on right now." Finally, you can acknowledge the reasonableness of the request while saying no: "What you are asking of me doesn't seem like much, but my plate is so full right now that I've made a promise to myself to say no to absolutely anything else for a while."

In addition to plugging the big drains, perfectionist mothers will feel more sexual energy when they cut back on the small but cumulative depletions that characterize fear- and guilt-based mothering.

Overcoming Perfectionism

Many maternal perfectionists believe that mothers who take time for themselves are either selfish or have perfect husbands or relatives who allow them their me-only time. Undoubtedly, some of the women who delegate and/or say no *are* selfish, and some of them *do* have very involved husbands. But not most!

Women who make it a point to have time for themselves have an entirely different understanding of how the world works. They refuse to internalize impossible expectations. For example, they base their self-assessment of mothering on realistic standards. They expect that mistakes come with the territory. They tolerate grumbling from their husbands when they know darn well they're entitled to some time off.

In contrast, certain worldviews allow guilt and perfectionism to flourish. The following exercises are designed to help you recognize and replace mistaken beliefs about mothering that are preventing you from making room for your own needs. This approach is based on the cognitive therapy model developed by Aaron Beck and popularized by David Burns. First applied to depression, the model notes that automatic negative thoughts and mistaken schemes contribute to low self-esteem and unhappiness. It's a way of conceptualizing the truism that we're all capable of being our own worst enemies. This model is now very popular in psychotherapy and has been applied to everything from unhappy marriages to obsessive-compulsive disorder. The goal is to harness your own common sense to fight self-defeating misperceptions and mistaken conclusions.

The following are some core beliefs about mothering that contribute to burnout:

1. "I must be a perfect mother."
2. "Doing what I want is selfish."
3. "I cannot make mistakes."
4. "My own standards can exceed everyone else's standards for mothering."

Your list may look just like this, or you may have your own list of core beliefs about what you expect from yourself. To quiet the twin demons of guilt and perfectionism, you will want to replace these schemas with more realistic ones.

The following will help you to replace these mistaken beliefs with more logical ideas. Pay special attention to modifying all-or-nothing (disaster-or-triumph) thinking about mothering.

"I must be a perfect mother."

More realistic schema: "While it is important to do my best as a mother, it is only possible to do the best that I can. I am capable of providing the good-enough mothering that will help my children become happy, healthy, responsible adults. Perfect mothering is a myth, and I have the power to refuse to believe in fairy tales."

"Doing what I want is selfish."

More realistic schema: "It's hard to find time for myself, and my children may ask for more than I choose to give. I know that when I'm relaxed and energetic, everyone benefits. I know that when I'm refreshed, I do my best work as a mom. I know that making time for sexuality is good for everyone."

"I cannot make mistakes."

More realistic schema: "Mistakes are not necessarily catastrophic, and they don't mean I'm a defective mother. All competent mothers make mistakes from time to time, and sometimes we learn the most from mistakes. When my kids see me handle my own imperfections, they learn how to do that in their own lives."

"My own standards can exceed everyone else's standards for mothering."

More realistic schema: "Although I operate on the assumption that I'll feel relaxed only if I meet my high standards, the truth is that my energy is drained by trying to do better than everyone else. It isn't fair or realistic to demand more of myself than I do of others."

If this doesn't immediately sink in, keep at it. The following techniques help you continue the process of thinking your way to more realistic mothering standards:

1. Put in writing that these are attitudes and not fact ("I believe I must be a perfect mother, but others do not believe in perfect mothering").
2. Spend a week writing down every time you catch yourself mentally or verbally expressing maternal perfectionism.
3. Generate a list of evidence that supports or refutes your core belief. Force yourself to list reasons why you might be mistaken.
4. Create your own list of affirmations or use a book of affirmations. Prayer and proverbs may serve the same purpose.

5. Consider seeing a professional therapist to strengthen self-esteem about mothering, especially if you were raised by a dysfunctional mother. The moms who are toughest on themselves are those who were insufficiently nurtured. They're incredibly vigilant about the risk of history repeating itself. Locate a therapist with specific cognitive therapy skills. Ask if she's trained and oriented to help you build your confidence using this approach.

6. Find a perfectionist-mom buddy and commit to kicking the habit together. Call each other once a week to report an imperfection, and help each other recognize the very good in the not perfect.

7. Laugh it off. Read Anne Lamott, Erma Bombeck, and Vicki Iovine, the goddesses of finding humor in the impossible profession of motherhood.

Mothering from Abundance

The emotion that underlies mothering dominated by perfectionism and its shadow, guilt, is fear. Fear as a basis for mothering may be traced to lack of good role models ("just don't let me do *that*"), a lifetime of criticism, or a generally anxious view of the world. Fear as a basis for mothering is terribly exhausting, yet often invisible. Fears may be ill-defined: If I'm not a perfect mother, something terrible will happen to my children. Fears may be highly specific: If I take time for myself, my children might not know how much I love them. Fear is based in scarcity, a core belief that you are at imminent risk of running out of what you need.

A huge shift in how you and your children interact takes place when you abandon fear and scarcity in favor of joy and abundance.

The very same interaction has an entirely different emotional tone. For example, making cookies for the Halloween party in a fear-based system entails worrying about what the teacher or other mothers will think, hoping your son appreciates the effort, and redoing "mistakes." Making those cookies in an abundance-based system that recognizes that kids like cookies allows you to laugh instead of cringe when your son puts three eyes on the pumpkin or proudly slops on the frosting. It transforms an action from one intended to ward off criticism by producing a perfect product to a process that is naturally enjoyable for you and your son.

Take a look at the basis of your own mothering. Can you find other examples in which fear is the foundation? Spend a day noticing every interaction with your child: Is it fear-based or abundance-based? When your preschooler dresses herself in plaids and stripes, is your first impulse to smile, or is it to insist that she change lest someone think you dropped the ball? When your eight-year-old plays goalie in soccer, are you proud of his courage or terrified that he'll lose the game for the team? When your adolescent comes home from a dance, do you anticipate that she had fun or worry that no one asked her to dance? Tuning in to what proportion of your mothering is motivated by fear or scarcity as opposed to joy or abundance may be enough to get you redirected.

If not, try the following steps.

1. Banish the audience. (They probably aren't there anyway.)
2. Focus on the process, not the outcome. (Your son may grow up with pleasant memories of helping Mommy in the kitchen, but he surely will never remember what the cookies looked like.)

3. Spend a week identifying each and every joyful aspect of your mothering tasks. (Does the fabric softener smell great? Can you relish the extra fifteen minutes you got to spend relaxing together before dinner on a night when traffic was light? Did you notice the beautiful illustrations in the book you read to your child?)

4. List what abundant emotional assets you have to share with your child. (Is your mother's "closet" stuffed full of creativity? Predictability? Safety? Soothing? Unconditional support? Humor? Values? Spirituality?)

5. List all the other people who contribute to your child's positive experience of the world. (Remember: It *does* take a village to raise a child. Who's in your village?)

Just Do It

A day of sexy self-care may translate into a boost in libido for a moderately stressed-out mom. The truly depleted may find that it takes much longer to recharge. If you are seriously burned out, give self-care at least three months to see the link between sex drive and overall energy.

If you recognize that the key issue for you sexually is depletion, stay with this step until you have mastered it. A therapist might help you get unstuck, and there are many great self-help books on the issue. Perhaps you have as many self-care books as you do diet books sitting on your shelf. If so, dust one off now! If you need some recommendations, here are some that I think are especially well done:

Breathnach, Sarah Ban. *Simple Abundance: A Daybook of Comfort and Joy.* New York: Warner, 1995.

Basco, Monica Ramirez. *Never Good Enough: Freeing Yourself from the Chains of Perfectionism.* New York: Free Press, 1999.

Domar, Alice, and Henry Dreher. *Self-Nurture: Learning to Care for Yourself as Effectively as You Care for Everyone Else.* New York: Penguin, 2001.

Placksin, Sally. *Mothering the New Mother: Women's Feelings and Needs After Childbirth, a Support and Resource Guide.* New York: Newmarket Press, 2000.

Affirmation

"When traveling with small children, please apply your own oxygen mask before assisting others."
—Every major airline in the country!

Step Three: Disarm the Internal Censor

"At virtually every stage of female development, girls and women receive confusing, and at times, contradictory messages concerning their bodies, their behavior, and their sexuality."

—Sandra Leiblum, Ph.D., Foreword, *Women's Sexuality Across the Lifespan*

- In the absence of supportive and accurate information, many women have a harsh internal critic that judges their sexuality.
- In contrast to the myths about wild sex in other people's bedrooms, most Americans are highly conventional in their sexual relationships. However, unconventional sexual practices are not rare or weird. You are the best—and should be the only—judge of what is sexually appealing in your own bedroom.
- A key step to reinvigorating your sexual intimacy is to turn down the internal censor.

A woman's internal critic and her internal censor are inextricably linked. The internal critic is your automatic faultfinder. The censor keeps a tight rein on sexual exploration. Both stand in the way of great sex.

Women rarely discuss sex practices with their girlfriends, doctors, therapists, sexual partners, or sisters. In the absence of information, we are left to draw our own conclusions about where we fit into the cultural scripts for what's "normal" and what's "sexy." Often, we are left with cultural caricatures, which give us impossibly contradictory guidelines. Without the facts, we are subject to pressure to conform to stereotypes of what constitutes "acceptable" female sexuality. Without the facts, we often feel that we fail to measure up, that our perceived deficiencies are uniquely our own.

Confusing cultural messages about female sexuality can be difficult enough pre-kids. Unfortunately, now we have a whole new set of cultural directives that tell us to be Nice Girls simply because we are moms.

One doesn't associate "sexy" with "soccer mom." You don't make out in the backseat of a minivan. Movies, novels, and television shows almost never depict loving, responsible, devoted mothers as sexually active and assertive. Media images haven't really moved forward from the days of Laura Petrie in her own twin bed. The rare exceptions in the media to the absence of sexuality in good mothers' lives are portrayals of divorced mothers: Michelle Pfeiffer in the movie *One Fine Day*, Selma Ward in the television series *Once and Again*. The fact that sexiness is reserved for divorced mothers just reinforces the message that sex, motherhood, and marriage are incompatible.

Without accurate or supportive cultural information about sexuality, we end up having one-way conversations in our heads. These internal monologues about sexuality are usually harsh. One person's internal critic may be telling her that she is a total pervert for her fantasies; another's internal critic may be telling her she's frigid or sexually repressed. Some warn you about your partner's response, certain that he'll think you're not a nice person.

The internal critical messages are often irrationally of the "damned if you do, and damned if you don't" type: Those fantasies are perverted *and* you're really a boring sex partner, for example. The critic is part censor, trying to convince you that you're expected to meet the community standards for moms having sex. The censor practically shouts at you to stop thinking those naughty thoughts, stay inside the lines.

One problem with the harsh internal critic, besides the fact that it is likely to keep you from exploring your own natural curiosity, is that you never get an opposing view. If you find it extremely embarrassing or awkward to talk with your partner or friends about sexuality, the critic is the *only* voice you hear. Cultural mythology about hot sex in other people's bedrooms just amplifies the critical voice that claims you're doomed/boring/perverted/all of the above.

In this step, I'll help you disarm the critic in three stages. The three stages are: believe that you're okay if you're highly conventional, believe that you're okay if you're not, and banish the censor.

Disarm the Critic: Believe That You're Okay

First, we'll refute the internal critic that says everyone else has a wilder sex life than you. Many women find it very helpful to know what is actually happening in other people's bedrooms. If you feel at all dissatisfied with your sex life, or your husband does, you may find comfort in knowing that those myths about mind-blowing sex just don't hold water. Most people have highly conventional sex and not nearly as often as one assumes.

Unfortunately, the most comprehensive and scientifically sound survey of sexual practices in America did not address the specific impact of motherhood.[1] Oops. Yes, invisibility of the sexual mom is a cultural problem even among the cultural critics. Nonetheless, I cite

---

[1]This study compared sexual practices and attitudes of married couples with those of single and cohabitating couples, but did not distinguish between married couples with and without children in the home.

their statistics on marriage as the closest approximation we have for married couples *with* children. Since an unrelated study found that only 6 percent of couples noticed a more satisfying sexual relationship after childbirth, we can also assume that statistics on married couples are actually the "best-case scenario" for married couples with children. That said, the following data are quite clear that *sex in America is conventional.*[2]

- Ninety-five percent of Americans' last partnered sexual activity was vaginal intercourse.
- Ninety-five percent of Americans usually or always have vaginal intercourse when they make love. Approximately 1 in 5 women report also receiving or giving oral sex the last time they made love.
- Most adults make love between four and eight times per month, whether they are married or living together, younger than twenty-five years old or older than fifty, religiously conservative or religiously unaffiliated, highly educated or a high school dropout, white or persons of color, and/or male or female.
- Most married people have sex a few times per month or less, although approximately 40 percent have sex two or more times per week.
- Among men and women alike, vaginal intercourse has the highest appeal among sexual practices.
- The majority of men and women between the ages of eighteen and fifty-nine report using a vibrator as unappealing.
- No women describe forcing or being forced to do something sexually as "very appealing."

[2]Robert T. Michael, John H. Gagnon, Edward O. Laumann, and Gina Kolata, *Sex in America: A Definitive Survey* (New York: Warner Books, 1995).

Use these findings to remind your internal critic that vanilla is the flavor enjoyed—emphasis on *enjoyed*—by most Americans.

Next, Remind the Critic That Someone (Else?) on Your Block Is Doing Something Unconventional

Kinky is definitely in the eye of the beholder, but many of us have greeted our own natural curiosity and sexual fantasies with disapproval and harsh labels. For example, although women do not find being forced to do something sexually appealing, fantasies of willing sexual surrender or submission are exceptionally common and normal, though often harshly self-labeled. Here I want to help you disarm the internal critic that claims you're supposed to be schoolmarmish in the bedroom.

There are solid data that prove that *nonconventional sexual practices are common.*

- One in five women have tried anal intercourse at some time in their lives.
- Forty percent of women report masturbating in the last year (including those with an available sexual partner).
- Two thirds of women have given oral sex in their lifetime.
- Three quarters of women have received oral sex in their lifetime.
- One in six women report that using a dildo or vibrator is appealing.

Use these data to remind your critic that so-called normal sexual practices fall under a very big umbrella.

Finally, Banish the Censor

Moms have so many "shoulds" and "should nots" ruling their lives. One is that moms should not explore their own sexual creativity. The fact is, parents or not, all sexually active humans have sexual fantasies, desires, and impulses. Many of us turn these off automatically, feeling shameful, perverted, or convinced that happily partnered women shouldn't go there. Turning down the volume on the internal censor will free up your own sexual imagination and creativity, which is bound to be best suited for you.

Using the same cognitive techniques discussed in Step Two, you can actively overcome your sexual reticence. Don't expect a major personality change. You probably won't suddenly start dreaming up plot lines for *Sex in the City*. Instead, expect a two-stage process. The first step is to suspend disbelief. The second is to discover that you are glad that you did so.

The steps that follow all involve making changes in what you say and do about lovemaking. My belief is that you've already taken your level of boldness just to your natural comfort zone. I'm going to ask you to move a little further. Start with the least-threatening idea. As you wander into new territory, you will find that it gets easier and easier. The idea of sexual innovation will become something that makes sense, and this provides a positive feedback loop for further quieting of the censor. "Not-me" becomes "me," but only by making the decision to open the door to that possibility.

Think Your Censor Away
Become Aware of It
Mentally notice automatic thoughts in response to sexual novelty.

These thoughts are likely to be along the lines of "Ewwww," "Icky," "He'll think I'm a slut," "That's pervy," and/or "No self-respecting woman would do that." These are self-critical, labeling, emotionally "reasoned" beliefs that stand in your way. Though they flow automatically, they are not automatically correct. Never mistake sexual beliefs for sexual certainties, especially when it comes to value judgments about sexuality.

Notice Black-and-White Thinking
Examples of categorical thoughts include, "If it isn't vanilla, it's perverted," "I'm too old for that kind of thing," and "What's next: a French maid costume and a leather whip?" These thoughts replace legitimate hesitancy with sweeping judgments. They take the middle out to the extreme. Stay in the middle.

Stop Predicting the Future
Predictions of the future generally include dreadful consequences, such as "It won't work," "He'd be repulsed," "I'll feel trampy," "I would giggle too much," "I'd simply die if I tried that," or "I would make a complete fool of myself."

Instead, acknowledge that the unknown is uncertain and sometimes frightening but also potentially very rewarding.

Apply More Accurate Labels
Use your common sense to replace distorted beliefs with more reasonable statements. For example: "I'm not vulgar, I'm interesting," "I feel foolish, but I'm still willing to let myself be vulnerable," "I'm afraid he will judge me, but I also know that he accepts and loves me," "I feel like I would die of shame, but no one has ever actually expired from trying something new," or "My husband will overlook awkward mistakes."

Leap Before You Look

Stop overthinking this whole thing. Yes, you have a lifetime's social programming judging your every sexual move. None of those good girl/bad girl messages is fact. There are no critical observers in your bedroom. You can choose vulnerability, choose to trust your own good judgment of a marriage partner, choose to experience before you decide that something just isn't for you. Jump.

Identify What Really Belongs in the Bedroom

Every time your censor sends an alert, pay attention to the values underlying the alarm. Decide whether your censor (probably an ancient relic from your youth) is the best judge for you as an adult and as a member of a couple.

Negativity loves a vacuum, and the censor will thrive if you don't foster counteracting positive values. Your critic may have some very good points (for example, that it is wise to take care not to be ridiculed), but may exaggerate the dangers and thereby exclude important conflicting values. The positive values a negative censor may have set out to promote initially include security, consistency, and safety. Unfortunately, your negative censor also allows in fear of criticism, political correctness, invulnerability, certainty, and other judgments that do not belong in a passionate relationship.

One way to banish the censor is to invite in a different judge, a wise and kind jurist who believes the interested parties are in the best position to decide what is sexually appropriate in their bedroom. This judge doesn't mistake bravery for foolishness in a committed relationship.

Become conscious of the sexual values you want to honor in your relationship. This may be as easy as going "uh-huh" to the list that follows, or you may need to focus all your energy on one value at a time. A patient in my practice described a "star chart" she developed to encourage her preschooler to listen better. The big ear she drew on the chart was an important statement to her son: I value this. For the next week, she praised and encouraged any and all listening she noticed. Voilà! By the end of the week, his listening improved, because she made it the top priority that week. She anticipates a need for a tune-up down the road, because new habits can be hard to maintain.

Do likewise for yourself in strengthening your sexual values. You may wish to write on a mental or literal yellow Post-it note the value of the week on your own imaginary star chart. Zoom in on that value, in the bedroom and out of it. Choose from the adjacent list of values found in passionate parents. Their biggest "secret" is that their sexual values are also their relationship values.

Values Shared by Passionate Parents

1. attentiveness
2. appreciation
3. a sense of humor
4. communication
5. courage
6. flexibility
7. imagination
8. receptivity
9. trust
10. vulnerability

How do these values facilitate moving away from plain vanilla sex? First, they let you access your own sexual imagination. Replacing fear and self-criticism with courage and a sense of humor gives you per-

mission to explore what is already in your head. It means that when
you see something intriguing in a movie, for example, you replace an
automatic censoring message with permission to consider a new sexual idea.

Embracing receptivity lets you take advantage of your partner's
creativity. His sexual imagination is as interesting as yours, and consciously choosing receptivity over discomfort or habitual disapproval
gets you out of the routine. Bear in mind that even Dr. Seuss thinks
you should try green eggs and ham before deciding you don't like it!

Use these values to guide you through the remainder of this book.
Some suggestions may trigger the internal censor's disapproval.
Notice those times when your reflexive response is "no way." Don't
accept the automatic censure. Instead, ask yourself whether exploring a particular sexual idea is consistent with the values listed above.
If you really can't countenance a particular practice, don't do it. But
make clearheaded and conscious decisions about your own sexuality.

Work toward strengthening these values, both inside and outside
of the bedroom, and your censor will slink off in shame.

Affirmation
"Mistakes are part of the dues one pays for a full
life."
—Sophia Loren

Phase Two
UNLOCK YOUR SEXUAL POTENTIAL

In the next four steps, I will make some very specific suggestions for increasing the erotic tone of your lovemaking. But be assured of this: There is no aphrodisiac as powerful as the mind. It is sexy to be wanted, and sexy to want. It is sexy to make love with nothing more erotic than our bodies and our courage.

Unfortunately, after making love for years or even decades, many couples are locked in a sexual routine. While I am certain that someone out there is having wonderful sex while making love in exactly the same way each and every time, most of us find that enthusiasm lags in the face of sexual monotony.

How routinized is your love life? Do you make love between the hours of 10:12 and 10:27 P.M. every fifth night? Do you always know when he turns off the news and follows you into the bedroom that he's going to initiate sex? Will it start with 3.5 minutes of kissing, 4.5 minutes of breast caressing, then 6 minutes of penetration?

Do you climax exactly 57 percent of the time? No wonder sex has lost its appeal.

While many mothers realize that they're bored in the bedroom, and have a vague idea about fixing it eventually, it's all too easy to drop the matter. Some of the hesitancy is identity conflict, the belief that motherhood and great sex are inconsistent. Some of it is fatalism, the assumption that sex with the same person inevitably becomes boring. But most of the reluctance is that we're too embarrassed to take a risk, constrained by what we don't know.

Why shouldn't you feel awkward and tentative? Who in your life has ever transmitted approving, loving, nonjudgmental encouragement for developing your own sensuality? Who in your life has given you anything remotely resembling practical information about sexual pleasure? In other times, in other cultures, the community of women might instruct you in the ways of pleasure, just as they would impart information about raising children, weaning babies, cooking, or cultivating herbs. There is nothing "natural" about our post-Victorian silence as a female community.

What is natural is the capacity every mother has to have great sex. You can overcome miscommunication, shyness, dulled senses, thoughtless hurried sex, and inadequate sexual knowledge. I'll show you how.

Step Four addresses communication. You may have great communication skills within your family life but freeze in the bedroom. I'll help you find ways to let your partner know what you'd like, with your body and your words. Step Five is actively boosting your own natural libido and getting unstuck from the gridlock of a painful sexual overture. Step Six brings you back to the world of sexual mindfulness, by transforming sex from something you do half-heartedly to something you savor with full attention. Finally, in Step Seven, I'll help you explore your natural eroticism. You can have great sex just by unleashing the infinite possibilities of the human senses.

As you continue in this section, recognize that you have unlimited potential to be sexually passionate. Believing that you have, or can easily access, all the treasures of human sexuality will open the door to solutions that fit your personal identity. With knowledge and intent, you can reclaim your sexual destiny.

Step Four: Find Your Sexual Voice

"Courage is what it takes to stand up and speak; courage is also what it takes to sit down and listen."
—Winston Churchill

- Many couples find it difficult to talk about sexuality in a deep and meaningful way. Fighting about sex should not be mistaken for communication.
- It is perfectly understandable to find it difficult to talk about sexuality. But if you don't take the risk, you have no chance of gaining anything. If you do and flop, then you are no worse off than you were before.
- Sexual communication by nonverbal means may be the easiest way to begin expressing yourself.
- How you deliver the message greatly affects how it will be heard.

Many couples are like the Taylors, who find it tough to communicate in the bedroom.

Amy's husband wants to make love at least every other day. Amy would prefer to make love far less often, perhaps once every couple of weeks or so. Amy has noticed that if they haven't made love in the past week, Bob gives her "the silent treatment," sulking and disengaging from her attempts at conversation or shared activities. She wants peace, so she accepts Bob's sexual overture once or twice a week. Amy's reality is that she is "giving in" to Bob's greater libido by making love more often than feels natural. Bob's reality is that he is accommodating Amy's lower libido by not "pestering" Amy sexually.

Amy and Bob rarely talk about their sexual relationship, but when they do, Bob says, "What's wrong with you? You used to like sex. You're never too tired to go shopping with your friends, never too tired to talk on the phone with your mother, never too tired to paint your frigging fingernails. You're just too tired for me." Amy gets defensive: "You think sex is like a switch I could just turn on? Maybe that's true for you, but I'm not just some machine. You try spending a day with the kids and see if you're so hot to trot at the end of it."

When I talk with Amy and Bob about their sexual relationship, it's immediately clear that each wants to be judged "right." Amy asks me to give her statistics on how often couples her age make love, guessing from her girlfriends' wisecracks about their sex lives that she isn't atypical. Bob wants the statistics to support his sense of deprivation, to validate that he has a right to expect sex more often.

While the Taylors are stuck worshiping the God of I'm Right and You're Wrong, even couples without a defense-attack pattern to their conflicts have a difficult time opening up to discuss sexuality meaningfully. Some couples, such as Amy and Bob, *appear* to talk about their sexual relationship, but their fighting is just fighting, not true communication.

Many couples simply avoid discussing sex altogether. It doesn't get to the fighting stage, because "don't ask, don't tell" is the implicit agreement. Vanessa and James are typical expert dodgers: When James is in the mood to make love, he'll start massaging Vanessa's neck. If she is interested, she nuzzles up to him. If she isn't interested or has something else on her mind, she stands up abruptly and busies herself with household chores. Unlike Amy, Vanessa does not defensively respond to an unwanted overture with annoyance. But just like Amy and Bob, Vanessa and James sidestep genuine communication about those times that their sexual desires conflict.

What's the big deal about avoiding talking about sex? Every single time you choose silence over dialogue, you honor fear. You validate secrecy and shame. And it's not getting you what you think: Your sexual character and propriety have absolutely nothing to do with whether you talk about your sexual relationship.

Silence also fosters misunderstanding. James may take Vanessa's disinterest as personal rejection and feel hurt or confused by her clear, abrupt message of "no," when it turns out that Vanessa's preoccupied by a conflict at work. Or James may do the complete opposite: miss Vanessa's communication that she is indeed upset with him, never seeing the unstated connection between the frustration she has over his unpredictably late days at the office and her sense of closeness. Without clarity, couples are relying on mind reading, a very faulty system.

Obstacles to Sexual Communication

Several factors make it difficult to talk about sexuality with our most intimate partner. For starters, because we generally marry at the height of sexual passion, we're at risk of getting blindsided down the road. The newness of falling in love is such a powerful aphrodisiac that sexual communication isn't an issue at first. Early-relationship sex is usually great because it's early-relationship sex. By the time you need good sexual communication skills, you may be a tad lazy about what it takes to keep negotiating your inherent individual differences. You may already be used to thinking like a unified couple ("We like anchovies on our pizza, we're Democrats, and we have sex on Saturday nights") and unused to having any important areas of conflict that need work. When the important area that needs communication work is something that most people find inherently difficult to talk about—sex—taking the bull by the horns can be doubly hard.

You may have married with all sorts of conflicts anticipated: where to live, how to handle Thanksgiving and in-laws, and countless other issues of both style and substance. The potential erosion of passion, however, doesn't register on the radar. But as time passes, and life with children gets more complicated and hectic, sexual differences begin to appear. It's the rare couple that is perfectly sexually matched during the child-rearing years. Eventually, differences in pacing, preferred practices, and interest in introducing novelty emerge, sometimes at a point in the marriage when the couple believes the big issues are already resolved. When sexual differences become clear in a marriage, the conflict-resolution skills and intentionality that worked in the early-relationship negotiations may be in dire need of a tune-up.

Another major reason for difficulty talking is that our sexual self-esteem is usually rather fragile. Typically, sexuality is an area of great vulnerability. Most of us are eager to be sexually attractive, worried about being sexually pleasing, concerned that we compare unfavorably to our partner's past lovers, and apprehensive about being sexually rejected. We may be afraid that our fantasies are "weird" or anxious about being "frigid." Likewise, we may be terrified that our partners would be devastated by our concerns.

Additionally, many couples unwittingly ascribe to the romantic notion that deeply devoted couples intuitively know what each other wants. Somehow, needing to ask or tell seems like a betrayal of true love. A common mistaken belief about marriage is that the other partner will know what we want before we even say it, and that having to ask for something makes it less valuable once received. It's the wish for getting the perfect birthday present without giving any hints, the hope that he'll somehow know that you really want to go to your mother's for Easter this year, or the fantasy that he'll magically show up with takeout dinner at the end of a day of the terrible two's.

Alas, marital ESP is usually a very poor connection, and it's especially so in the bedroom. It's a myth, just like the myth that everyone else is having nothing but mind-blowing sex. Don't fault yourself for having the dream, but don't get stuck there, either.

Improving Sexual Communication

First, a few words about communication in general. Early in training, psychotherapists learn to understand verbal communication in terms of two key components: process and content. Process is how the message is delivered. Examples of process issues include timing, location, and circumstances. Content is the nature of the message. Examples of content include criticism, praise, fear, and self-disclosure. Issues of process can cloud content, such as when one of you brings up a touchy issue two minutes before dinner guests are due. Issues of content can distort process, such as when an issue is so painful that you circumvent it for eons before coming to the point.

Another framework for considering issues of communication is the verbal-nonverbal dichotomy. This is especially relevant for sexual communication, where much can be accomplished—or botched—by body language. Tuning in to content and process issues as well as what you say without words provides a blueprint for improving your sexual communication.

Although I'm not giving you permission to ignore the hard stuff, I'm all in favor of first approaching the problem from whichever angle is most comfortable (or, perhaps, the least uncomfortable). You can develop better sexual communication by working on strategies of process, or you can start with the specific content issues. You can decide to use words, or you can decide to communicate nonverbally. You can also reach for the stars and work on all fronts.

Sexual Communication: Nonverbal

Many women find that nonverbal communication is the easiest way to start. This will be true especially if you had a particularly strong gut reaction of "no way" to the idea of talking directly about sexuality. When my patient says, "I could never look him in the eye and talk about our sex life," I know that she's very uncomfortable, but I refuse to let her give up so easily. However certain you are that you couldn't talk openly about lovemaking with your partner, I discourage you from predicting the future. You may find that successful nonverbal communication opens a door that looks closed to you right now.

Nonverbal sexual communication is most useful for providing information about what feels good to you. He cannot possibly know what his touches are doing, or not doing, without useful feedback. Many women hesitate to provide nonverbal feedback because they underestimate the importance men place on being sexually pleasing to their partners. We don't have the corner market on other-orientation, and I give you my guarantee that your partner would like more, not less, feedback. Intimate couples derive pleasure from giving pleasure.

The first way to provide nonverbal feedback is by touch. You can do this one of two ways:

Direct his touch to the right spot(s). Take his fingertip and place it in the exact place that feels great, most commonly the clitoris. While I'm assuming that you know where the right spot is (either because you've brought yourself to climax before or been touched there[1]), I'm not assuming that the clitoris is your only erogenous area. Show him all the good places, perhaps during different acts of lovemaking. If you worry that this will seem implicitly critical to him, remind yourself of how different our bodies are. Even the smallest penis is easily located. If the shoe were on the other foot, wouldn't you like to know exactly where to caress?

In addition to showing him nonverbally where to touch, *show him how to touch you.* People tend to generalize from their own experience, but this can be faulty when it comes to male vs. female preferences for the intensity of pressure in a sexual touch. The clitoris has the equivalent number of nerves as the entire penis, meaning that millimeter for millimeter, the clitoris is far more sensitive than the penis, where nerves are dispersed over a larger area. Men often prefer a stronger pressure whereas women usually prefer a lighter caress. This is highly variable.

When using personal preferences to guide their touches, men may push or rub too hard, and women may not provide enough pressure. This is a potential pitfall of nonverbal communication. If your husband is pressing too hard, you may lighten your own caress in the hopes that he'll figure out that you want a lighter touch. If you are stroking too lightly, he may increase the pressure in the hopes that you will get *his* message. As with verbal communication, clarity is important. Rather than modifying your touch on *his* body to signal the intensity of caress that feels good to you, show him on *your* body. When he's pressing too hard, take his hand and demonstrate a lighter touch. If he's too light, apply a little pressure to his fingertip.

[1]If not, pick up either Lonnie Garfield Barbach, *For Yourself: The Fulfillment of Female Sexuality,* rev. ed. (New York: Signet, 2000); or Julia R. Heiman and Joseph Lopiccolo, *Becoming Orgasmic: A Sexual and Personal Growth Program for Women,* rev. ed. (New York: Fireside, 1988), and explore the self-touch exercises therein.

Once you've braved this, try to find the courage to show him exactly how much pressure you like at each of the sensitive parts of your body, which likely respond maximally to different levels of pressure. If you can, notice and then share with him the way in which your sensitivity changes as you get closer to climax. Typically, men enjoy a firmer touch as they near climax. Women may enjoy a progressively lighter touch, although firmer pressure at the moment of climax may be just the thing, usually followed by excessive sensitivity that can make postclimax touching painful.

Some men are unaware that good lubrication enhances clitoral pleasure in addition to facilitating intercourse. If you'd like more lubrication when he is touching you, and you have adequate moisture during foreplay, place his finger inside your vagina, then bring it up to your clitoris. Or have KY Jelly or Astroglide handy (available over the counter at a pharmacy) and apply some to his finger at the right moment.

Another very effective way to *communicate nonverbally is through sounds*. Some women enjoy moaning or sighing during lovemaking; others are terribly inhibited about the idea. If you saw the movie *When Harry Met Sally,* did you laugh or blush and squirm when Meg Ryan verbally mimicked a loud climax at the restaurant? Of course, even if you enjoy letting loose with sounds, the presence of children down the hall can inhibit just about anyone. Know that vocalization is an incredibly powerful way of providing positive reinforcement for the shy—it communicates praise, is not threatening to anyone's ego under any circumstances, and is clearly win-win for both partners. And read on to learn how to moan for your lover's ears only.

Overcoming the Inhibition

Perhaps you're thinking, "I could never moan during lovemaking." I hesitate to use the term "moaning" here, because that may have a horrifyingly negative connotation for some women, conjuring up images of being outrageously unladylike or primitive.

To some extent, this sense that lovemaking sounds are animalistic is an effect of Hollywood, which takes the image to the extreme. Just as everyone climaxes simultaneously in the movies, Real Women announce their orgasms to the entire neighborhood. What I'd ask that you consider is more of a murmur than a moan, or an expressive sigh.

Practice a quiet throaty sound right now. Start by making the sound you undoubtedly make often (outside the bedroom) that communicates "I don't think so" or "We'll see about that": "hmm." The sound is made with your throat, mouth closed, as you push air out quickly. Now use the exact same mechanics (i.e., mouth closed, pushing air across the vocal cords) but make a quiet murmured "mmm," as if you are enjoying your first delicious cup of coffee in the morning. That's it.

That sound is all it takes. Make it when your husband is touching you in a way that feels great, and he will repeat it. We all love praise. Making small murmurs that convey appreciation and approval will lead to more of what feels good.

What if the kids hear? First, you do not need to project—you're right next to each other, for heaven's sake. You can make a highly effective but modest sound that will not carry past a closed door. Convince yourself in your most protective mom mode that you can do this. You'll be more relaxed when the appropriate opportunity arises if you've tried this out loud. If you're still too anxious about the kids overhearing, put a sound between them and your bed. This could be a radio or boombox turned low, just inside the doorway. It could also be a white-noise machine, either one made to induce sleep in travelers and babies, or a fan, air purifier, or humidifier placed at the door.

And so what if the kids hear? If they're old enough to know what those sounds mean, they won't ask about it. If they're too young to understand, they may be frightened. Simply reassure them that what they heard was a sound that grown-ups make when they are touching one another in a special grown-up way. You'll all survive.

You may find that your comfort with expressing pleasure nonverbally increases as you try it. If your husband begins doing the same thing, you will see how delightful it is to get positive feedback. When the opportunity arises (no kids around), consider trying to consciously ratchet up the sound level of nonverbal feedback for a change.

Sexual Communication: Using Words

Attend to process issues first. This means pay more attention early on to how you deliver the message than you do to its content. Creating comfortable space with comfortable boundaries to talk about your sexual relationship will make the process easier for both of you. The following are some suggestions about what might work for you.

First, the Don'ts

Don't fight about sex while making love. That probably seems obvious, but it can easily happen if you don't see the fight coming. Avoid issues that might be painful or inflammatory during lovemaking. Topics that easily turn into an argument include frequency of lovemaking, performance issues, or bartering ("I'd be more interested in sex if you'd . . ."). Pick the right time, which is never in the middle of sex.

Don't accuse. Humans are hardwired to get defensive when we hear phrases including "you never . . . ," "you always . . . ," "you need to . . . ," "you shouldn't . . . ," "I wish you would just . . ." You get the point. Unfortunately, the natural tendency to flinch at "you" statements directly collides with female reluctance to make "I" statements. Women often have difficulty completing the phrases "I would really like . . ." and "I want . . ." We've been raised to accommodate and please. Many women feel so uncomfortable asking for what they want that they tend to phrase requests as entitlements, demands, or accusations of deprivation by their partner. Rather than admit that they have wants that someone important hasn't provided, it is tempting to express the *want* in terms of a *need* that the other has withheld.

Amy is like many readers who wish that cuddling and kissing didn't always have to lead to intercourse. Because she wants to please her husband, she has accommodated by refraining from affectionate overtures unless she's definitely ready for complete lovemaking. Lately, she's been more aware that she isn't happy with this arrangement and that she'd like to have the option of more nonsexual touching without intercourse when she feels like it. Notice the difference between the statements "You never just want to cuddle anymore," or "You know I need more affection than you do," and "I would love to cuddle without necessarily making love more often." The latter statement lacks accusation, but it requires Amy to acknowledge her wishes and preferences.

Don't escalate antagonism. Examples of conflict multipliers include:
    Categorizing your partner: "You're a sex maniac . . ."
        Substitute: "We have really different ideas about how often to make love . . ."
    Magnifying the issues: "You never . . . ," "You always . . ."

> *Substitute: "Right now, I'm feeling . . . [stay limited to the present issue]"*

Exaggerating: "I've asked a million times for . . . ," "For once, why can't I have it my way? . . ."

> *Substitute: "I feel really certain that I'd be more energetic for sex if I weren't feeling so drained by the end of the day."*

Precipitating counterattack: "I've done everything I can to . . ."

> *Substitute: "We seem stuck on this issue."*

Criticizing: "How about thinking about me for a change?"

> *Substitute: "Here's how it feels from my angle."*

Using sarcasm: "Well isn't that sexy . . ."

> *Substitute: "I'm more likely to get turned on by . . ."*

Mind reading: "I know you say that, but what you're really thinking is . . ."

> *Substitute: "Let me clarify. You're saying that you feel . . . is that right?"*

Negative body language: Eye rolling, skeptical facial expressions, shaking your head while he talks.

> *Substitute: Be aware of maintaining "open" body language: relaxed posture, arms and legs uncrossed, shoulders open, neutral facial expression.*

Don't bargain for sexual intimacy. Sex as a reward for good behavior, in exchange for something else in the relationship, and/or withholding sex as punishment or payback is painful to acknowledge but common. Take an honest look. Are there times when you wish he'd connect the dots as to what leads you to say yes or no? If so, you may be attempting to communicate by a sexual bargain. Could you choose a different, more effective communication strategy?

Playful "exchanges" are not the same as bargaining. I'm not referring to a flirtatious "keep telling me how great I look and I promise to curl your toes when we get home." Bargaining rests in anger and frustration. In contrast, a playful invitation—"make me want you"—is a great strategy for a libido mismatch.

Next, the Do's

Set the ideal time and place. Rather than arguing in bed, when sexual vulnerability for one or both of you is at its greatest, select a time and place when you're likely to start out feeling in control. Empathy and generosity flow from strength, and both spouses will be kinder and more receptive when starting out on solid ground.

Some specifics that may help couples discuss sexuality include:

- Start a discussion about sexuality only when there is no chance of interruption, especially by children. If the phone rings, let it go unanswered.
- Consider talking on the phone, or in the car when you're both looking forward. Not making direct eye contact may reduce self-consciousness as well as aggression.
- Set a time limit. After five or ten minutes, negativity often escalates. It's better to stop too quickly than too late. Reschedule another time for unfinished business.
- Establish the right to bail out. Make this explicit from the outset as follows: "Talking about our sex life is new for us. This feels a bit scary, and yet it's very important. It will be more productive if we both can agree to bail out if needed. Let's start by deciding that either one of us can call a time-out if we're just too uncomfortable to continue, with no questions asked. We'd arrange to

come back to the topic when we're feeling calmer or less defensive. Is that agreeable to you?"

It is crucial to have a safe boundary without encouraging stonewalling. Stopping a *specific* discussion due to discomfort or an awareness of high emotional reactivity should not end the *general* conversation. Reschedule, and proceed with caution, but do proceed.

Talk to your husband like he's company. Be polite, be generous, be open, be gentle. All too often, our partner is the only person in the world to whom we fail to extend common courtesy. Ask for clarification, stay calm and receptive, tune in to how he is likely to receive your message.

If you catch yourself escalating into anger and accusation, imagine that instead of fighting about sex with your husband, you're discussing a neighbor's request to borrow your leaf blower. If you're arguing loudly, categorizing, and magnifying, for example, imagine that instead of saying "I'm too tired to have sex because you're such a jerk and you never help me" to your husband, you're shouting, "I'm not loaning you the leaf blower because you're such a jerk and you never return anything" to your neighbor. You'd probably tell your neighbor a simple, calm "No, I can't lend you the leaf blower." Or you'd lower your volume, explain the problem ("I need it next week, and I know it's sometimes hard for you to find the time to get things back"), and invite joint problem solving. You wouldn't pour out everything that you've stored up, mentioning the time two years ago when his dog got loose and scared your kids, etc. Your husband deserves no less.

Make a good opening move. Statistically speaking, women are more likely to initiate discussion of highly charged items. As John

Gottman points out, that also means we're more likely to begin a conversation harshly, and "discussions invariably end on the same note they begin."[2] Anxiety about sexual communication may contribute to a harsh opening statement.

If you feel comfortable initiating a face-to-face dialogue about your sexual relationship, and all you need is a nudge in the right direction, great. If not, consider one of the following strategies:

- Give him written information as an opener. Start with Appendix A, "Sexual Advice for Dads." Or try an article in a women's magazine or some other pages from this book. The idea is that there is comfort in knowing that you're not the only ones experiencing a sexual problem. If you can't imagine opening the discussion directly, consider adding a yellow Post-it note that says, "Look this over and let's talk about it." Or if it's a new sexual practice or idea you'd like to try, attach a flirty invitation, such as "I bet this writer would really have had something to say if she'd had *you* to check this out with."

- Send him e-mail. Many couples find that e-mail is a terrific way to defuse hot-button topics. Consider attaching a Web site address or Internet article that opens the door.[3] Choose something that lets both of you know you're not alone. Invite him to take time before responding to your e-mail, and do likewise with your response to his response, so that you don't shoot from the hip and get a round of flaming e-mail started.

- Write him an old-fashioned pen-and-paper letter. This is an effective way to communicate your individual concerns while re-

[2]John M. Gottman and Nan Silver, *The Seven Principles for Making Marriage Work* (New York: Three Rivers Press, 2000), p. 161.

[3]Try: http://redbook.women.com/rb/marriage/ or http://www.oxygen.com/topics/sex/index.html or http://www.ivillage.com/relationships/.

ducing the anxiety or unintended hostility that can make it hard to initiate a difficult conversation. You can write and rewrite your letter until you're satisfied with how and what you've said.

Notice the good stuff. You catch more flies with honey. Praise the effort, praise the outcome, praise him. You may be so angry that you don't feel much like applauding what you've missed for so long. Try anyway, lest you win the battle but lose the war. Being right can be the most hollow of victories. Staying authentic and specific without being smarmy allows you to reap the benefits of praise without feeling like he got away with something. "That felt great last night when you gave me a back rub and I fell off to sleep" will be more effective than "Thanks for not pushing sex last night, for a change," and no less authentic than "So big deal—for once I get some cuddling without having to put out."

Be Brave

Making highly specific verbal suggestions can be terribly intimidating. There is no easy way out here—you're simply going to have to gut it out. You have nothing to lose if you fail and much to gain. Planning specific words to use in advance will help you find courage.

If the issue is . . .	Try . . .
You feel rushed.	"Let's make love really slowly tonight."
You want him to spend more time in a particular way or at a particular spot.	"Promise me you'll never stop doing that" when he is in the middle of something great.

If the issue is . . .	Try . . .
He sometimes quits before you've climaxed.	"I'm right on the edge."
You're bored with the routine.	"Could we try a little experiment tonight?"
You want to stop before intercourse.	"Could we pick this up right here another time?" (More about intercourse vs. erotic touching in Step Six.)
He is missing the right spot.	"I'll be putty in your hands if you just move an inch up." Or move his touch to the right area.
You're exhausted.	"I know sex energizes you, but I'm just feeling too tired to give lovemaking my full attention."
You'd like more oral sex.	"I'm turned on just thinking about having your mouth on me."

Be Generous

Being generous means taking the first step to ask for what you want. Get out of gridlock and go first. There is another important aspect of generosity: demonstrate good listening. One of the most effective ways to communicate is to set the example of receptivity to constructive input. Model what you'd like for him to do: "What feels best—this, or this?" Ask him, "Is there a way I could touch you that would feel even better for you?" Or "When I'm doing something you really enjoy, would you let me know?" You might ask, "Is there anything I usually do that you'd just as soon skip?" If you think you're reading his body language, or his nonverbal messages, ask, "Am I reading you right that you really like this?" Taking the first step can be a powerful invitation for him to respond in kind. As Yogi Berra said, "You can observe a lot just by watchin'." Make it comfortable for him to observe sexual vulnerability and communication.

You may find that the questions themselves are sexy. Even if you've been married fifteen years, you can have the kind of conversation that new lovers might have. How exciting!

Tolerate Initial Discomfort

Expect that the first attempts at improved sexual communication will be extremely awkward. Feeling awkward is icky but not deadly. Embarrassment is not terminal. You can tolerate the discomfort. Hopeful silence hasn't worked, and you would have found an indirect way already if you could have. Getting through the discomfort is worth the tremendous benefit that follows. Not only will your sex life improve, you may find that your courage brings you to a new, deeper level of emotional intimacy.

Affirmation
"Decide that you are strong enough to handle the risk."
—Phillip C. McGraw, *Relationship Rescue*

Step Five: Awaken Your Erotic Interest

> Q: How do you get a woman to stop having sex with you?
> A: You marry her.
>
> —Anonymous

- Threats to boosting sex drive include power struggles, guilt, and comparison sex.
- Elements that promote libido include romance, receptivity, and intentionality.
- Real moms can recharge their libidos by becoming more playful and more strategic in negotiating sex.

Chances are, you've heard the "joke" about how women stop wanting sex the minute they're married. I know I have: on the radio, on the Internet, in magazines, and in real life. Perhaps, like me, you don't see the humor. My response is usually to cringe or to counter irritably, "Yeah, well how do you get a man to stop romancing a woman? You marry him." Or I want to say, "Well, you push a seven-pound object through your sex organ and see how enthusiastic you feel about sex." In other words, I jump right into the finger-pointing fray.

But offensive jokes sometimes bear a grain of truth. In this joke I see a common situation in America's bedrooms. It captures the fact that sexual mismatch is a difficult subject to talk about directly. As with ethnic "humor," the jokes mask the teller's discomfort. And my response ("it's not us, it's you guys") crystallizes the potential for a power struggle over who's at fault.

The "joke" invites us to frame the issue of low(er) maternal sex drive in terms of fault. Someone must be wrong, and someone else must be the victim. Neither the joke nor the understandable defensive counterattack will be useful in any way. Rather than labeling the low-drive spouse as the "problem," it is helpful to recognize that this is a couple issue often grounded in the social realities of family life. As you work through this chapter, consciously reject self-blame or blame from your partner.

In addition to fault finding, there are three common difficulties that interfere with increasing your libido. While interrelated, these difficulties can be categorized as power struggles over frequency of sex, guilt, and comparison sex. All three are ineffective strategies for increasing libido in couples characterized by a mismatch in sexual drive.

Power Struggles

Power struggles are exceedingly common when a woman has less sexual interest than her partner.[1] As in any power struggle, the partners are battling to be declared the victor, and conflict resolution is not the goal. A couple having a power struggle over sex isn't working together to negotiate how often to have sex; each partner wants to "win." Sexual labels ("frigid," "overgrown adolescent") are quickly applied, and each partner walks away from the struggle feeling misunderstood and angry. Any compromise feels like surrender.

Low sex drive may be the result of power imbalance, when the low-drive partner feels that the *only* thing she's in charge of is sex. If a husband is extremely authoritarian, sex may be the only situation in which she can assert herself. Or the marriage may be egalitarian in most ways except for sex, when a woman feels disempowered to say

[1] If your situation is reversed, adapt these comments and suggestions accordingly.

no to lovemaking. Alternatively, the higher-sex-drive partner seems like the one without any power, as he tries harder and harder to do something, anything, that will make his partner sexually receptive.

Since the first obstacle to improving a libido mismatch is the power struggle, it is important to figure out whether this power struggle is specific to sex or part of a bigger problem. Relationships plagued by control and authority issues are characterized by battles over how money is spent, what activities children are permitted, which church is correct, and who chooses vacation spots. No issue is spared. Spouses in marriages burdened by power struggles virtually always fight over sex, too. If you have a power struggle over how often you have sex, and you also have control issues about everything from what the kids eat for breakfast to how often his mother comes to visit, you will need to address the larger issue before you can resolve the sexual power struggle.[2] Attempting to isolate the sexual issue in the midst of significant control and inequality issues is doomed to fail; at best, it merely relocates the battlefield.

It is easier to overcome an isolated power struggle that is the result of mismatched libidos. In such a marriage, most decisions are made peacefully, and partners resolve conflict outside the bedroom with a general atmosphere of equal participation, with each being heard and respected. An isolated sexual power struggle most typically involves initiating and refusing, a contest for who determines whether to have sex. Sexual power struggles may be linked to a single issue of greater importance to the low-libido partner. For example, Lisa and Carlos have both noticed that they make love more when Carlos has been helping out around the house. To Lisa, it seems only natural that she feels more loving when Carlos acts like a caretaking partner; to

---

[2]Apply the suggestions in Step Four to improve communication about nonsexual issues, or see Michael P. Nichols, *The Lost Art of Listening: How Learning to Listen Can Improve Relationships* (New York: Guilford Press, 1995).

Carlos, it seems that he needs to jump through certain hoops in order to get sex. At a deeper but perhaps invisible level, Lisa may withhold participation in sex while Carlos withholds participation in household chores.

Guilt

For some women, the issue isn't a power struggle—it's just plain guilt. Patti, thirty-six, and a mother of three, may speak for you:

> "I think my husband would have a heart attack if I ever initiated making love. I am fine once we get going— I usually get into it, and I can almost always have an orgasm, but I swear, I just never go to bed thinking about sex. Even if it's been great the last time, the very next time my reaction to him is always 'Again? Do we have to?' Then the guilt kicks in, and I feel like a terrible wife if I say no."

Patti's guilt indicates that she experiences her lack of sexual enthusiasm as a personal weakness, something she's selfishly withholding from her husband. She labels herself as defective and feels that she is letting her husband down. Women like Patti often notice that they have a sense of shame that their husbands got a "raw deal."

Guilt is not the exclusive property of the low-drive spouse. Patti's husband may feel guilty about "imposing" on his wife and may wonder if his libido, or even his technique, is the problem. He wouldn't push her to go to a movie she doesn't want to see, but he finds himself cajoling her into having sex, which leaves him feeling guilty.

Comparison Sex

Comparison sex often accompanies guilt and power struggles. Comparison sex goes like this: "It isn't fair that we never have sex. It's not normal to have sex only a few times a month, so I know I'm justified to want sex more often." Or "My girlfriends all talk about how they're so exhausted they just want to fall asleep the second they get into bed, so I know I'm just like everybody else."

Comparison sex is a dead end. There is no set standard of what constitutes "normal" sexual frequency. Normative—how often other couples make love—doesn't constitute "normal." For example, it's normative in the United States to have brown hair. Red hair is rarer but no less normal. Likewise, whether the neighbors are doing it more or less often than you and your husband has absolutely nothing to do with whether you, or they, are having great sex.

Comparison sex doesn't work: Statistics are not a useful way to motivate a low-drive spouse to want more sex or a high-drive spouse to want less. It isn't relevant to your sexual relationship. In fact, low sex drive is the most common concern of people seeking treatment at a sex therapy clinic.

You are not alone.

Understand Each Other

One of the most useful ways to unlock a power struggle is to get a better understanding of how the issue of initiating and refusing sex feels to the other partner. Taking blame and guilt out of the equation, work to listen to how the other experiences the libido mismatch. Remove hurtful labels, which often include the following: selfish, cold, pushy, passive-aggressive, withholding, frigid, or freakish.

Instead, conceptualize the issue of sexual overtures and refusals using the labels of "constructive" and "ineffective." You can exchange written information or, if you feel bold and safe enough, you can role-play. Be open to laughing at yourself, but be sure that your category of "ineffective" is free of mockery. The low-drive spouse should make a list (or role-play as described further in this section) of ineffective sexual overtures. For example, "C'mon honey, it's been two weeks, give a guy a break," is an ineffective overture, but he may feel that you are being sarcastic if you characterize his overture in this manner. Substitute a more general description of what is an ineffective overture, such as "references to how long it's been" or "entitlement." A common ineffective strategy is male communication of wanting to make love on the basis of *his desire for his own sexual pleasure* when she would like to know that *he desires her.*

At the same time, you simply must provide your husband with constructive suggestions, whatever they might be for you. He cannot read your mind. Some examples might include "You look so great that I really want to get my hands all over you," or "I can't stop thinking about how soft your skin feels next to mine." You may want to be more general: "letting me know you think I'm attractive," or "making me feel special."

You also need to understand how he experiences your refusal. Ask him to write a list of ineffective refusals. Be open to considering that what seem to you neutral, nonthreatening no's may be very painful for him. For example, he may feel as hurt by "not tonight," as he does by "Are you obsessed with sex?" A common, ineffective strategy for female refusal is experienced as a global sexual rejection, when he would like to know that *you find him sexually attractive* but *don't want sex* right then. Ask him to generate a list of ways you could say no more constructively. If that seems too difficult, try some of the words listed in the box.

Saying No to Sex Lovingly and Constructively

Affirm that you love and desire your partner in general but are not in the mood for sex at that specific moment. Examples include:

- "Hmm, I'm sort of tired tonight, but would you ask me again tomorrow?"
- "Wow, that's a really great invitation, but I'm going to take a rain check."
- "That thing you're doing feels wonderful. Could I request an instant replay another time?"
- "Last time we made love was so nice that I can understand why you want sex right now. I had some other things planned for after the kids fell asleep. Can we wait until I can give you my full attention?"
- "Honey, the fact that I am not in the mood right now means that the sexiest man in America isn't going to get lucky tonight."

Some couples find it helpful to write the lists together, especially if done playfully. A sex or marriage therapist might have a couple do this in a session so that she/he could provide a safe and supportive environment for what can be a hot-button topic. If you feel able to try this on your own, go for it, but don't force it. Don't hold it against your husband if he refuses, because few men will find this even slightly appealing. If you think your husband might be game, tell him, "Hey, I read about this idea where we each role-play one another asking for or saying no to sex. The idea is to become more aware of how the other partner feels during that exchange. Does that sound useful to you?" Drop it if he responds with anything other than "Sure!"

If you are both comfortable with this exercise, bear in mind that the goal is to increase each partner's awareness of how the other interprets verbal and nonverbal responses to an invitation to make love. Each of you must assume that how the message is received by the other is "true" in the larger sense. Do not get derailed arguing over the intent of either the initiator or the refuser. If he feels sexually rejected, don't argue the fine points of your meaning. Say it differently next time. Likewise, don't let him argue you out of what you're feeling about his overture. Be specific about what you'd like next time he asks to make love, and stand firm.

Another goal of this information exchange is to detoxify the issue. All couples have times when one or the other doesn't want to have sex. Couples with a low-drive spouse are either unaware or can't remember that negotiating sex doesn't have to be hurtful. Generating nonhurtful messages outside the bedroom will help you stay emotionally connected at times of sexual disconnection.

Overcoming Guilt

Like guilt about declining anything you don't really want, feeling guilty about saying no to sex is self-defeating. A reluctant sexual partner is not what your husband wants, and saying yes when you mean no always comes back to haunt you. The more sex you agree to under duress, the more you don't want sex. You simply must stop having guilt sex and trust that you can increase your sexual interest by other means. Part of your guilt about saying no is based on the way you say no, and taking the steps described above will alleviate guilt. A relationship-affirming no goes a long way toward alleviating guilt because authenticity in your sexual relationship preserves, not harms, your intimacy.

Guilt about saying no to sex is often based in a mistaken belief about male sexuality. Many of us grew up being warned by our elders about the dangerous need for release of male sexual desire. We were warned about "teasing," or putting men (or boys at the time) in a horrible state of sexual frustration that they would be unable to control. The residue of these messages in marriage may be that it is cruel to say no to sex, or that husbands will inevitably stray if not sexually satisfied at home.

You have an obligation to negotiate sexual frequency with loving sensitivity. You have an obligation to pay attention to your relationship, including your sexual relationship.

You don't have an obligation to have sex under duress.

Your husband has an alternative sexual outlet that he's probably already using: masturbation. Most men masturbate, including some very sexually satisfied married men (and, of course, women). Masturbation is a very different sexual experience than making love, but it certainly provides sexual release. It may be uncomfortable to imagine your husband masturbating, but until you stop feeling guilty, your libido is likely to flounder. Understanding that masturbation is an option also alleviates libido-killing comparison sex.

What Does Boost Sex Drive?

In addition to relaxation, as described in Step Two, sex drive for mothers requires three other basics: romance, receptivity, and intentionality.

I know it's preaching to the choir to point out that women thrive on romance. What may be less obvious, however, are the ways to inject romance into your relationship. Whatever your plan has been, if you aren't getting enough romance, you need a new strategy. It's been said that people often come to therapy seeking permission to keep doing the thing they're doing. The same is probably true for advice books. The hard thing about changing is that what you've been doing seems so sensible. It's the other person's response that seems to be the problem. The good news is that while you can't change other people, you can change yourself in ways that *invite* changes in others.

Many women have tried asking, demanding, or begging for more romance. You may have longed for romance but never spoken out loud about it. You may have tried to get your husband to read about Venus and Mars. Consider the following alternative strategies:

Go First

Become more romantic. Remember all those things you did early in the relationship to let him know that you thought he was special? Romance is about details and small meaningful gestures. Becoming more romantic may mean leaving him voice mail that he'll pick up when he gets to work, buying him token gifts, bringing him a rose, telling him he smells great, touching him more frequently. Avoid confusing mothering with romance: Don't expect that organizing his sock drawer or making his favorite meal is setting the example you want. (If he reciprocates by finally hanging that picture you wanted in the hall, it won't do much for your libido.)

In addition to romancing him, regard yourself as a romantic person. Get candles for the bedroom, own at least one lacy piece of lingerie, and resuscitate old habits. What did you do when you were first dating? Surely you didn't wear old sweatpants or floss your teeth in front of him. The comfortable ease of familiarity is a wonderful aspect of marriage, but the intentionality of female mating rituals is a wonderful aspect of sexuality, for both of you. Balance the sweats with perfume.

Increase Nonsexual Touching

Typically, a woman whose libido lags behind her husband's stops kissing, holding hands, and hugging. This is often due to a fear that he will mistake your intent or become sexually aroused and end up pressuring you to make love. There isn't a way out of this that doesn't involve discussing the issue. Tell him that you intend to increase your physical affection, that you believe this will increase your libido in the long run, and that you are concerned that he might feel more sexually frustrated. Ask for license and reassurance that you can try this.

You may be concerned that your husband will not respond well to all this communicating. You may worry that he will shut down or resent the talking. If you're married to a guy who would rather have surgery without anesthesia than talk about relationships, choose your battles wisely. Meet him halfway by not bringing up every issue, but don't accept never as an appropriate standard of marital communication. Acknowledge that he hates this girl stuff and remind him that the goal of the communication is better sex, something you're both interested in.

Accentuate the Positive

Make a genuine effort to notice and appreciate any and all romantic acts by your husband, however small. Just as you can become invisible, so he can become invisible to you. Heighten your awareness of the gestures that you've taken for granted. Tell him what pleases you, and use the word "romantic" as in "It's so romantic to have a husband who _____." A single instance of praise is more a more potent reinforcement than ninety-nine complaints of not getting what you hoped for.

If you feel romantically neglected, you may find this unpleasant.

Do it anyway. If you need to, set some boundaries for a time frame ("I'll give this two months, then I'm quitting if he doesn't change"), but throw yourself into it. If you simply cannot find a single romantic act to praise, gingerly notice romantic acts by others. This is delicate, because "Look how sweet that guy is being to her," can easily be heard as "unlike you, who never does anything romantic." The way the message is delivered greatly influences how it is received, and reception is everything here. Try instead, "I know it's just a movie, but wasn't it so romantic when . . ."

Ask for What You Want

Without gender stereotyping too much, it's useful to acknowledge that male and female communication styles often differ. A girlfriend who says "I need your support about my divorce" doesn't need to list: a) let me vent, b) invite me to dinner on holidays, c) reassure me that I'll date again. You know what she wants the instant you put your mind to it.

But if you ask your husband to "be more romantic," he may just not get it. Be direct and specific in your requests, carefully eliminating entitlement and resentment from the communication. Assume that he hasn't done so lately because he had an informational deficit, not because he's an insensitive jerk.

When an occasion for a gift approaches, tell him that you'd be so pleased with a bracelet or a sexy nightgown rather than ask for a vague "romantic present this time." Ask him to stop and pick up fresh flowers and then tell him how charming it is to see him walk through the door with a bouquet, even though it was your idea in the first place. Request that he make reservations at a romantic restaurant and couple the request with the local newspaper's Valentine's Day restaurant guide.

Help him succeed.

Receptivity

A profoundly simple change that boosts libido is becoming more receptive. Receptivity means that "maybe" precedes "no." Receptivity means staying open to the possibility that you might become more sexually interested, even if sex is the farthest thing from your mind at the moment. Receptivity requires two preexisting components: freedom to say no at any stage and increased nonsexual touching.

Many women in long-term relationships simply do not experience a spontaneous need for sexual release. In men, the influence of testosterone makes sex drive far less contextual. Female sex drive is typically dependent on emotional intimacy needs and is highly situational. Further complicating matters, sexual arousal occurs in response to different triggers and at different paces in men and women. The most common trigger for men is visual. If your husband tends to pounce on you as you're coming out of the shower, you understand this phenomenon. For women, the most common trigger is tactile, meaning that we often need to begin making love before we know whether we're in the mood. The slower pace of arousal in women means that we need more time to decide, but it also means that we may wish to stop at a point when our partner is far less inclined to do so.

The importance of touch for female sexual arousal is the primary reason why receptivity combined with increased nonsexual touching is critical for libido enhancement. It simply must be acceptable to kiss passionately, rub each other's backs, and yet be allowed to say no at times. Embracing receptivity allows a woman to explore the possibility of sexual arousal without "committing" to a decision to make love. This incredibly significant change in a couple's sexual dance will be easier with strong sexual communication skills. See page 128 for some suggested ways to say "no."

The converse side of female receptivity to "yes" is male receptivity to "no." In many couples, sex gets better when women don't say no too quickly *and* men take no more readily. Many women report that male receptivity to no is very affirming sexually, because they feel more wanted as an individual. When a woman's partner pushes for sex, she is likely to feel that he wants sex, not sex with her. As one woman said, "I used to feel like what he really cared about was that part of my body. This way, I feel like he really cares about me, what I want as a person. I'm not just an outlet to plug into."

It is a myth of male sexuality that men are all-or-none, that sexual frustration is a terrible thing to do to someone you love. This myth often brings couples to the gridlock in which the wife is unreceptive unless she already knows that she is willing to make love. Is this an assumption you've made? Ask your husband whether he'd be willing to risk more maybe's as you explore this. He may not confess, but chances are pretty good he's had one or more unconsummated erections already today. Your wish to spare him arousal may not be what he prefers.

Intentionality: Think Sexy Thoughts

This is a good time to remember that the brain is the major human sex organ. Indeed, our brains are often so filled with kid stuff that we literally push sexuality out of our consciousness. Our bodies are often utilitarian: our breasts are for nursing, our hips for toting toddlers, our laps for sitting. Our minds are for lists: school supplies, lesson schedules, work projects, grocery items. Just as we need to increase our awareness of the sensual aspects of our bodies, we need to honor our sensual minds, too.

Thinking sexually used to come naturally. It doesn't now, so you need to make it conscious. One reason why our male partners are often more sexually charged is simply because they have many more spontaneous sexual thoughts (perhaps due to the influence of testosterone). They are also less likely to scold themselves for having them, less likely to feel that noticing an attractive person is disloyal, and less likely to worry about the inherent impracticality of a passing fantasy.

It might be useful to imagine your sexual mind as a part of your identity that has gone into hibernation. The best analogy I can make personally is to gourmet cooking. I used to make up recipes and shop for the freshest, most interesting ingredients on a regular basis. I went into a great grocery story anticipating a pleasurable cooking experience. Since becoming a mother, I cater to picky eaters, and time is a luxury. Now I look for quick, easy, and sure to please. Gorgeous cuts of fish, fresh herbs, lovely loaves of fresh bread go unnoticed as I head straight for the plain pasta section. On those occasions when I do intend to cook for pleasure, I have to enter the store with a completely different mind-set. I have to begin thinking creatively about cooking days in advance, since I can't be sure the inspiration will strike me at the store. I've gone from being a spontaneous cook to an intentional one.

Taking our sexual minds out of hibernation requires intentionality, too. We can't expect our sexuality to thrive in a dark closet in the basement. Becoming asexual in our minds is a downward spiral: The less we honor and integrate the non-mommy self, the more the mommy becomes our only identity.

The next several chapters will explore some very particular real-mom ways of revamping our sexual minds. You may not need a sexual cookbook, but rather simply to decide to open the closet door of your sexual mind. If you can reach back in your own history to find what has worked for you, great. Others do best with some specific suggestions. See the adjacent box for some ideas.

Take Charge of Getting in the Mood

1. Wake up in the morning and decide to think about sex that day. (Make it like National Stop Smoking Day—pick a day and do it.) If you can, set a reminder on your electronic organizer or watch to beep every hour. When the beep sounds, think about sex.

2. Plan something specific you'd like to ask your husband to do to your body.

3. Remember a really great time the two of you had in bed.

4. Write your husband a sexy e-mail.

5. Give your husband a real kiss, the kind your kids may not have seen before. Make it last one minute. (I promise that this will not scar your children for life, even if they're old enough to be disgusted. Ignore their claims of being grossed out.)

6. While you're eating, play footsie under the table with your husband.

7. Touch him five times during dinner.

8. Whisper in his ear that you want to make love very slowly tonight.

9. Watch a romantic video while the kids have their own movie going.

10. Read sexy stuff (see Step Eight).

Ideally, incorporate those ideas that intrigue you into a day set aside for revving your libido, as described previously in Step Two. Don't just allow your sexual self to peer out of the dark basement closet, let her take charge of the house. Like any skill left neglected or newly acquired, temporarily immersing yourself at the beginning is the best first step toward mastery.

Get *Him* Thinking Sexually

Some women find that a little whimsy goes a long way. One difference between boyfriends and husbands is that boyfriends seduce, husbands expect.

Give your husband the following assignment: to make you want sex by tomorrow evening (if you're feeling really bold, ask him to make you beg). Tell him that in the words of singer Joan Armatrading, you're "open to persuasion." This playfully gives him the responsibility for romancing you, for becoming mindful about *his* role as the seducer. Being the initiator isn't the same as being the seducer. Men get tired of always being the initiator, the one who risks rejection or maybe even pleads. If you aren't yet ready to be the one who initiates sex, ask him to seduce you. It's win-win. He gets out of the supplicant role; you get the attention you appreciate and a glimpse of your old boyfriend. It may be a far more effective way to increase his attentiveness to pleasing you than asking for more romance.

Take Charge

Many women with faltering libidos assume that something external needs to happen in order for them to want sex again. While it is possible that there is a chemical basis for low libido (including antidepressant medications and/or perimenopausal or menopausal testosterone deficiency; see Step Ten), most of the time low libido is a gradually acquired response to boring, entitled, fatigued, hurried, or unemotional sex. In other words, it's a bad habit. Getting out of the habit of not having sex very often requires taking individual responsibility for becoming more sexually awake again at the same time that you take steps to make your sexual relationship more interesting, inviting, refreshed, and engaged. Stop waiting for it to come back. Make your libido a gift you insist on having for yourself.

Affirmation
> The Possible's slow fuse is lit
> By the Imagination.
> —Emily Dickinson

Step Six: Cultivate Sexual Mindfulness

"It is remarkable how easily and insensibly we fall into a
particular route, and make a beaten track for ourselves."
—Henry David Thoreau

- Any couple can increase sexual intimacy by increasing
  sexual engagement and attentiveness.
- Mindful lovemaking transforms sexuality from a destination to a state of erotic being.
- The key step to becoming more mindful in the bedroom is staying present in the erotic moment.

Many Americans—rushed, driven, pressured, hassled, and drained—
have turned to Eastern philosophy and spirituality to help them find
meaning. We're frustrated by a cultural heritage that values the goal,
not the journey. We literally focus so much of our attention on
achieving particular outcomes that we are always in motion, never
where we want to be.

Savor the present. Slow down. Get comfortable being. Stop racing
around. This message has tremendous value for American mothers,
both inside and outside of the bedroom. Inside the bedroom, savor-
ing the present means becoming more mindful about sexuality. Sex
can be just like taking a walk: It can be a powerful spiritual experience, or it can be monotonous. What determines the quality of the
experience isn't the destination. It's the process, the how you go
rather than the where.

> **Married sex is hurried sex.**
>
> • Dating couples are four times more likely to take an hour or more when making love than married couples.
> • Married couples are more likely than dating couples to devote fifteen minutes or less to sex.

The human mind can experience only one conscious thought at a time. However, we are typically so mentally busy that we jump from one thought to another, which makes it seem as if we are thinking about several things all at once. Indeed, our culture demands multitasking: Capable mothers rarely do one thing at a time. Not only do we never learn to stay in a relaxed yet engaged place for very long, we actually train ourselves to juggle ever more.

Passion and multitasking are natural enemies. Passion, by definition, is singular and consuming. One way to work your way back to more passionate lovemaking is to practice being absorbed by lovemaking itself. As you and your partner get more focused on your sexual relationship, your pleasure will increase. As French thinker Simone Weil said, "The highest ecstasy is the attention at its fullest."

Mindful sex means paying attention, engaging, giving, and staying open. It means letting go of performance anxiety, distraction, history, and body self-hatred. If becoming mindful in your lovemaking seems easy, keep practicing until you realize how hard it is! If becoming mindful in your lovemaking seems very difficult, you're on the right track.

The concept of mindful sex is very simple. The goal of mindfulness in the context of lovemaking is to transform doing or performing into being—experiencing. The application is where the challenge lies. Take the following suggestions in small steps. Select one or two ideas and practice those for a while. It's absolutely contrary to the point of this chapter to tackle these ideas as if they were a "to-do" list or a set of skills to be mastered.

I'm asking you to shift your thinking about lovemaking and invite your partner to do likewise. Mindful lovemaking has no set end point, no gold star that tells you that you're done. Staying present, awake, and alive during lovemaking is like kindness or laughter in a marriage: There is always room for more.

Commit to Letting Go of Anxiety

Identify the sources of anxiety that accompany lovemaking. For many of us, body self-hatred is on the top of the list. For others, it's performance anxiety, which can include fear of disappointing our partner, falling short of an unrealistic standard, or anxiety about failing to climax. Another source of anxiety can be male sexual dysfunction, which can include fear that he'll climax too soon, not climax at all, or lose an erection.

Committing to letting go of anxiety in lovemaking means that you decide to give fear less control. You cannot tell yourself to stop worrying any more than you can stop thinking about elephants the minute I mention elephants. What you can do is make the promise in principle to loosen worry's grip.

Some women find that heightened awareness alone helps release sexual anxiety. When you become aware of an anxious feeling or thought, label the thought. Mentally note, for example, "Here is that worry about whether I'll climax this time." Labeling the worry immediately makes it less powerful because you're acknowledging that this is a fear, not a fact. Don't judge or criticize the worry. Remind yourself that you choose to let go of this worry: "I've decided to let my worry about climaxing leave now." Shift your attention back to your physical self. If you are able to fully engage your present mind in lovemaking, the anxiety will leave on its own.

Others find that mental imagery helps send sexual anxiety on its way. First, as you become aware of discomfort, imagine the worry as words on a banner trailing behind a small airplane. Create the image in your mind of the banner floating across your mind's eye, lightly waving in the breeze. Mentally watch the plane enter and leave your field of vision. Alternatively, you might find visualizing a cue word helps you become more present, such as "notice." You may need to repeat this a few times.

Body self-hatred is a tough demon to banish. Try to detoxify it by acknowledging that this is *your* issue—not his. Understand that your fear that he will be turned off by your body is a belief, not a fact. If he *is* criticizing your appearance during sex, you have a troubled marriage, because this is highly unusual husband behavior. They don't care. He is not thinking about your thighs or stretch marks or the bags under your eyes. Overwhelmingly, what does irritate men is our body preoccupation. Stop asking him for reassurance. Believe that he desires your imperfect body.

> ". . . in many, if not most situations, we each have the opportunity to 'show up' as ourselves regardless of weight."
> —*Deb Burgard, Ph.D., www.bodypositive.com*
>
> This site is a fabulous resource for body size acceptance.

Create Sacred Sexual Space

Churches, synagogues, mosques, and temples are beautiful places. Do we need an environment of beauty to access a higher power? Of course not, but it doesn't hurt. All religions encourage us to separate the spiritual from the mundane, to consecrate the space in which we search for a deeper connection. Saying a blessing before a Sabbath dinner, wearing one's finest suit to church on Sunday morning, settling onto a beautifully crafted meditation pillow are ways in which we remind ourselves to prepare for something special. Mindful sex is special, too, and your physical environment should reflect this before you make love.

A parent's bedroom is usually anything but sacred. There may be dust balls under the bed, old breast milk stains on the tattered pillowcase, Beanie Babies under the covers, or even sleeping children. Creating sacred sexual space for parents isn't like it used to be when you were first dating, and you could just cram all the papers into a closet and quickly make your bed before your boyfriend arrived. Creating sacred sexual space now means creating a feasible but deliberate ritual that invites an extraordinary experience.

An important aspect of sacred sexual space is having a sexual boundary (see Step One). Some specific rituals that you might use to metaphorically put on your Sunday best include having a special quilt you throw over the everyday covers that comes out of the drawer only for lovemaking, burning incense or a scented candle, changing the sheets before lovemaking, using linen spray (such as The Good Home Company's Pure Grass sheet spray, available at www.beauty.com and Nordstrom's), having a clean sleeping bag that you throw down on the bathroom floor (the only room in the house with a functioning lock), or turning on a white-noise machine that muffles bedroom sounds.

Give More of What You Want

Turning to non-Western spirituality, try the following: Give more of what you fear you lack, what you feel you can't possibly spare. Stop avoiding the fire of anxiety or deprivation: Walk right into it. Your perspective will change. In the bedroom, this translates into a paradoxical approach—immersing yourself in that which you fear:

If you are distracted by body self-hatred, notice and notice again your husband's physical attractiveness. Pay extra attention to the features that you find appealing. Tell him. Turn the lights on.

If you are anxious about him climaxing too quickly, take more time to make love.

If you are anxious about not climaxing yourself, decide to make love to him unilaterally—leave your clothes on and don't let him touch you.

If you are anxious about being sexually inadequate, do nothing at all. Insist that he make love to you.

Use these as learning opportunities. Expect to find that you were unable to predict the outcome, and stay open to learning new information. You may find the unexpected. Noticing the beauty of the curve in his jawline or the arch of his foot, for example, may help you make room for acknowledging your own beauty.

Practice Staying Present in the Moment

For many mothers, making love is a rare opportunity to slow down. It is common for distracting thoughts to pop into your busy head. You may have noticed similar patterns when you get your hair cut, soak in the tub, or even wait at a stoplight. Mundane thoughts immediately float into consciousness: forgotten permission slips, the trip to the bank you neglected, a phone call you must make.

As is true for anxious thoughts, it isn't possible to simply will these thoughts away, nor is it a good practice to ignore them. Instead, when kissing, touching, or making love, become aware of nonsexual thoughts as they appear. Pay more, not less, attention to how often your mind wanders during lovemaking.

Next, as nonsexual thoughts occur, gently redirect your focus toward your physical and emotional sensations. Consciously shift your attention to your body and notice where and how your husband is touching you. Tune in to every detail. Change your mental narrative to an observation of what is happening within your body. Direct your attention to your own actions, too. Notice where your hand is drawn, what his skin feels like, how he looks and smells and tastes.

A key aspect of staying present is letting go of predicting or controlling the future. Become mindful of how often your thoughts move ahead. Whether your thoughts run ahead to worries (how tired you'll be in the morning if you don't get to sleep soon) or pleasant thoughts (what a terrific climax you're about to have), increase your consciousness about this obstacle to staying in the present moment.

Eliminate the Goal

This step is the most "present" approach of all: stop thinking about orgasm, period. I can hear you and your husband protesting! I am not advocating becoming nonorgasmic or joining the Tantric once-a-year orgasm club. What I mean is eliminating consciousness about climax while erotically pleasuring one another. Orgasm is a natural response to sexual stimulation and pleasure. Worrying about it is counterproductive. Additionally, delaying orgasm by a few days usually intensifies the next climax. Your body has a memory, and it will remember the craving for release.

Reframe: You didn't fail by not climaxing, you gained an intensified experience for the future.

Here is a radical suggestion: substitute attention to your partner's nongenital body. Cultivate nonorgasmic erotic pleasure. Stop imagining that lovemaking has a beginning, middle, and end. Try to conceptualize lovemaking as a series of physical pleasures, some of which will include climax, some of which will not.

Mindful sex means not hurrying to the finish line. The next time you have ten minutes for a quickie, decide to touch one another erotically but not climax. Substitute ten minutes of nipple caressing or take a steamy shower together. Remember that sexual tension is great once in a while. It can be terribly exciting to be frustrated, eager for the next encounter.

Anticipation is erotic.

Instead of viewing lovemaking as a predictable event that occurs all at one time and in one place, conceptualize sexuality as a sequence of related physical pleasures. Intentionally caress each other without having intercourse for as long as you can stand it (days or weeks). If your husband is reluctant, help him understand that this is very different than days or weeks of not having sex the way you've been not having sex. This is not having intercourse while becoming much more sexually intimate and involved.

Start with more intense kissing. Can you even remember the last time you kissed for fifteen minutes at one time? On the following night, take ten minutes to explore each other's hands. Aim for daily sensual contact. If five minutes is all you have, so be it. More is better, but some is good, too. Gradually intensify the sensuality of your touches. Move from the feet and hands to caressing one another's inner thighs. Delay involving genital contact for as long as possible.

Even then, try to avoid bringing each other to climax for several days (although by this time, you'll be itching for release).

When you absolutely cannot stand it another moment, give in and make love. I guarantee better sex. How can I be so sure? In part, because anticipation is a powerful, uniquely human aphrodisiac. It's the pleasure of smelling fresh bread baking, waiting to see your favorite performer in concert, knowing that tomorrow is Christmas morning.

This approach offers more than heightened anticipation. Every single part of your body has erotic potential. Every bit of your skin contains nerves that can be aroused sexually. Certain body areas are intensely enervated, and we naturally gravitate toward those areas, such as the nipples, clitoris, and penis, especially when time is precious. Focused mindful touching reprograms and awakens forgotten areas. You literally uncover a world of erotic potential just by paying attention to different areas, while temporarily avoiding erotic hot spots. Try to defer touching each other's genitals until you feel ready to burst with desire, ideally several weeks into this process. Even then, avoid orgasm and intercourse for a bit longer, if possible.

Why avoid sexual intercourse initially? If you feel like making love, shouldn't you do so? Isn't that the point? For starters, unless the goal of orgasm is made off limits, habit will take over. You're just too used to lovemaking leading to a particular outcome. Also, you are finding out about your body's erotic potential, and physiologically, you will not tap into all that is possible unless you shut down "overused" areas temporarily.

This approach is also an incredibly powerful lesson in appreciating the potential for lovemaking to be a connected chain with links made up of a series of sexual experiences over time. Many parents have completely compartmentalized sexuality, putting sex entirely out of our minds and bodies until and only when engaging in the specific activity of sexual intercourse. As women, we may be aware of this as a longing for more "affection." As couples, we experience this as sexual boredom. By increasing erotic touching with the specific intent to defer intercourse, we immerse ourselves in an erotically energized world, transforming our recent notion of sex as something one is too tired for to a source of energy. (More specifics are covered in Step Seven.)

Cultivate All Five Senses

Becoming aware of each individual sensation bridges the mind-body gap in lovemaking. Often, we overemphasize the sense of touch and fail to notice and savor other sensory experiences in lovemaking. We may even take tactile experiences for granted, mindlessly going through the motions. For a change, try to notice the extraordinary in the ordinary.

Start by distinguishing types of touch, including how his body feels to your fingertips and how his touches feel against your skin. Become conscious of the nuances of touch: notice how his lips feel against your neck, how it differs when he strokes your skin lightly or firmly. Observe how sensations change geographically: What are you experiencing as he caresses your labia? And how does it change as he moves toward your clitoris? Find new tactile input: his heartbeat, the feeling of his boxers against his penis.

Also cultivate your attention to other forms of sensory input: look, listen, taste, and smell. Concentrate on a single sensation, tapping into the marvelous details that you simply forgot to notice. Listen, for example, to the sounds each of you makes. When your mind wanders, pull your attention back to hearing his breathing, noticing murmurs, becoming aware of how your own breathing sounds at the moment. This is covered in greater depth in the next chapter.

Practice Generosity

Actively nourish loving and kind ways of "seeing" your partner. Become aware of unkind sexual assumptions that you make, and substitute a more generous attitude. The following are examples of how to give him the benefit of the doubt.

If he wants to make love after a fight:

Instead of assuming he's "a typical man who still wants to have sex no matter what," consider whether he wants to make love to reconnect emotionally.

If he's rushing you in bed:

Instead of assuming he's "selfish," consider whether he's really turned on by you at that moment.

If he's doing the same thing every time you make love:

Instead of assuming he's dull, consider whether he's found what he thinks is a sure way to bring you pleasure.

If he's pushing to try something that feels kinky:

Instead of assuming he finds you boring in bed, consider whether he trusts the marriage enough to explore new territory.

Practice generosity and mindfulness outside the bedroom, too. It is absolutely erotic to have your lover reach over and fill your half-empty water glass at dinner. Being noticed is captivating. Noticing your partner is seductive. Tune in to his space and pay generous attention to his body outside the bedroom. Take his towel and finish drying him off. When you're putting lotion on your hands, rub some into his, too. Feed him a bite off your plate at a restaurant.

Practice Thankfulness

Actively let your partner know what feels good to you. Tell him what feels good both when it is happening and later. A reference outside the bedroom to something that happened inside the bedroom is not only very sexy but also likely to increase his interest in repeating something that you enjoyed.

Developing sexual gratitude is much like other forms of spiritual gratitude: You must practice, practice, practice. If you've ever tried keeping a gratitude journal, you know how paying attention to the things that bring you joy changes your world. It is awkward at first, especially if you feel scared or mad or hurt.

Start by developing sexual thankfulness as if you were making love for the very first time. When you were seventeen and making out in the backseat of your boyfriend's car, you forgot to notice how amazingly wonderful the human body is. Find the miraculous now. Contemplate the enormous wonder of something as mundane as holding hands. We have hands for so many useful things, but, truly, isn't it just incredible that two human beings can communicate trust, affection, connection by intertwining their fingers? How about kissing? Could anything be as marvelous as the lips?

Keep Practicing

Many of the suggestions in this chapter will feel clumsy and stilted at the beginning. Although we often assume that great sex is innate, the only thing about sex that is "natural" is the procreative science, not the art. You're a parent: You've already reproduced. Now is the time to explore the art of lovemaking. Many other cultures view lovemaking as something one learns, studies, reads about, practices, and gets better at over time. Mindful sex is a habit that must be practiced consciously to become second nature.

Without repeated practice, you probably won't ever get comfortable with this approach. Avoiding orgasms, even temporarily, will seem ridiculous if you quit before achieving body knowledge of pleasurable erotic contact. Changing the fundamental assumptions of how you make love is like taking up tennis for the first time. You look silly in blindingly white gym shoes, your backstroke is pathetic, and you want to give up. But, as with tennis, once it clicks, once your body understands the flow of the sport, you're hooked. You don't need to keep repeating the awkward first steps; eventually it all becomes effortless.

Suspend disbelief about "training" for mindful sexuality. It may take just one trial of abstaining from intercourse and orgasm-directed lovemaking to reap the benefits, to permanently become more absorbed in lovemaking as the ultimate here-and-now experience. Or you may find that this approach is worth revisiting as needed: at times of sexual disconnection, such as the birth of a new baby, an illness in the family, or an emotional impasse in the marriage. Any time you feel that the centrality of the present moment has slipped away from your lovemaking, start at the beginning again and work your way back through a disciplined approach to a relaxed mindfulness.

Affirmation

"In sex, there is nowhere to go but right here, right now. All we need to do is focus on this moment with our lover, without selfishness or thought."
—Philip Toshio Sudo, *Zen Sex*

Step Seven: Explore Erotic Geography

> "Our senses also crave novelty. Any change alerts them, and they send a signal to the brain. If there is no change, no novelty, they doze and register little or nothing."
>
> —Diane Ackerman, *Anatomy of the Senses*

- Enhancement of all of the body senses will dramatically intensify your physical intimacy.
- Erotic geography is easy to learn and apply. Your body and his body are infinitely pleasurable.
- Harnessing the power of sexual trust is the secret weapon of committed couples.

Sex with a new boyfriend is full of novelty. Sex with the father of your children offers much more. You get to have sex with someone who cares deeply about your pleasure, who has come to know your sexual triggers, your body's best spots, your likes and dislikes. This can translate directly into more pleasurable sex. For example, studies show that married women are more likely to climax during lovemaking than single women. Familiarity can be a boon for great sex.

Unfortunately, familiarity can also become monotonous. Great sex makes the best of both: It integrates sexual discovery with learned experience. Great sex uses the foundation of the old as it welcomes the new. Welcoming the new takes knowledge and a commitment to pursue new ways of bringing pleasure to oneself and one's partner.

There's an old joke that goes, How many psychiatrists does it take to change a lightbulb? One, but the lightbulb has to really want to change. You have to want to change, have to want to rejuvenate your sex life more than you want to stay in your comfortable shell. That's really all it takes: the decision to suffer through the initial awkwardness. Bear the discomfort, and you'll be happy with the results. If you're really stuck here, go back and work some more on banishing the internal censor.

Cultivating the Senses

Take your first step toward sexual innovation at the edge of safe territory. You will find it easiest to make relatively modest changes, to venture ever so slightly outside the familiar. The art of making love is largely about intentionality, mindfulness, and making the ordinary extraordinary. In Step Six, I encouraged you to become more aware of the sensory experiences in your current lovemaking. Now I'm asking you to start spicing up your love life by actively accentuating the novelty and enjoyment of the five basic senses during lovemaking.

Some specific suggestions for deepening each of the five sensations (sight, hearing, smell, taste, and touch) follow. Take one sense at a time and find what feels comfortable and exciting for you. Don't get overwhelmed trying to do everything all at once!

The Visual Sense

Throw a red scarf over a nightstand light.
Make love during the day.
Open your eyes during lovemaking. Watch your partner's face.
Pull the covers back so that he can watch you as you caress his
　　body.
Get a gorgeous nightgown for yourself.

Get great boxers, or boxer-briefs, for him.

Keep one loose item of clothing on: a camisole, an oversized sweatshirt, his Oxford shirt. Have him keep an item of clothing on.

Make love wearing only high heels.

Apply one of your child's temporary tattoo flowers to your inner thigh or just below your navel.

The Auditory Sense

Listen to his breathing. Try to synchronize your breathing.

Notice how he expresses pleasure.

Become aware of the sounds you make.

Play Brazilian music in the background.

Make a cassette tape of your lovemaking sounds. You might feel most comfortable if you trash it the second it's done (a pair of scissors to cut the tape is all it takes to childproof it), but you might find it exciting to put the tape on next time you make love.

Put your ear to his chest and listen to his heartbeat. Observe how it changes, communicating excitement.

The Olfactory Sense

Notice how his laundered shirt, his soap, his aftershave, his perspiration smell.

Add a nonfloral aroma, such as sandalwood incense or a patchouli candle.

Use scented massage oil, such as almond or citrus scents.

Have him apply lavender-based lotion to your skin. Breathe in
   the aroma.
An hour or two before lovemaking, tuck any of the following between the pillowcase and the bedspread: a fresh rose, a few
   sprigs of rosemary, mint leaves.

The Gustatory Sense

Find his naturally salty areas.
Sprinkle orange juice or champagne on his chest, then taste
   him.
Pop an Altoids peppermint in your mouth. After a few seconds,
   lodge it off to the side, then taste his nipples. If you're feeling
   very bold, try giving and receiving oral sex the Altoids way
   (don't use a cinnamon Altoids down there!).
Feed each other Chinese food while nearly naked in bed.

The Tactile Sense

Have him wash or brush your hair before lovemaking.
Introduce soft fabrics: silk pajamas, satin sheets.
Powder each other.
Pick your (noncotton) panties off the floor and run the fabric
   through the web of his toes, one by one (or use his silky box-
   ers).
Lather each other with soap (be sure not to get any inside your
   vagina; it can be irritating—stay external).
Hand him a feather (those big peacock-type feathers sold at im-
   port stores are especially soft).

Touch is perhaps the most erotic of the senses.[1] Ironically, however, the very power of highly erotic zones can end up contributing to boring sex. After years of making love together, many couples know exactly where to touch to maximize pleasure. But just as you fail to notice the pressure of your watch against your wrist after a few minutes, going for the gold each and every time can become humdrum. Touch serves as one of the body's major danger alarm systems. With repeated touch, interpreted by the brain as "no danger," the body eventually turns down awareness to a familiar touch, while increasing attentiveness to novel touches.

Even if you know that you'd like to diversify, chances are extremely good that no one ever told you where to touch, how to touch, or ways to explore being touched sexually. A wonderful scene in the 1999 woman-directed film, *Kama Sutra*, shows a courtesan teaching her students the fine points of erotic touching. I'd be hard-pressed to think of something one would be less likely to see in American culture. Because sharing erotic information is culturally taboo for "nice girls," expect that you'll feel somewhat clumsy at first and even a little silly. You will get the hang of it. Keep your sense of humor in the bedroom and don't take any of this too seriously.

You May Have Places You Don't Want Touched

There isn't an unerotic spot on the body, although there are certain areas some individuals find unappealing. If you or your partner are genuinely uncomfortable (that is, not merely bashful), don't go there. Sex is supposed to be fun, and never something to be endured.

[1] As an oversimplification, men tend to be especially sensitive to visual sexual stimuli, while women are most sensitive to tactile stimuli. Women are also generally more sensitive to auditory input than are men.

The area most commonly cited as sexually unappealing is the anal area. Some couples, however, find this to be one of the most sensitive and exciting areas, because the nerve supply is extremely dense and/or because the taboo itself is arousing. No one is right or wrong here. Some people find equally unappealing the feet, hairy armpits, and even the vaginal area, especially for oral sex. It is worth noting that women tend to underestimate how much men actually enjoy cunnilingus and/or the female aroma of vaginal secretions (another example where body self-consciousness is our issue, not theirs).

A final taboo is making love during menstruation. Some women are uncomfortable making love during their periods. Some use it as a handy excuse to say no. Except during first- or second-day cramps when you just don't feel well, there is no biological reason to abstain during the menses. You or your husband may be ill at ease about the messiness of it or find the concept itself distasteful. Some couples are comfortable touching and penetrating but avoid female oral sex during the menses. Other couples are completely unfazed by menstruation. Again, there isn't a right or wrong way to be. However, given how much difficulty parents have finding sexual opportunities, it seems a shame to have any limitation for as much as a week every month. Try using an over-the-counter product called Instead.[2] This is a rubber cup that holds menstrual flow out of the vagina. When you insert an Instead, you and your partner will not notice any menstrual blood.[3] This provides *no* birth control. If you use a diaphragm, you can accomplish both contraception and contain menstrual flow, but if you choose to bathe, do so before you insert the diaphragm

[2]Available at any pharmacy, usually next to the tampons and sanitary napkins.

[3]You might want to stick a dark-colored towel under your pelvis to catch any post-coital tinges of red in your secretions or his ejaculate, but don't expect more than a trace. If you're really self-conscious, a bath or shower after inserting the cup will wash away further traces of blood.

and contraceptive jelly, or simply wash off residual blood on the external genitalia after insertion, being careful not to wipe away the contraceptive jelly.

Erotic Geography

Knowledge is power, and sexual power is fun. Increasing your attention to your lover's erotic map is likely to enhance your sexual self-esteem, give you a pure sexual charge, and result in him paying more attention to your pleasure zones. If you open the door, he is very likely to respond in kind.

As a general rule, the more important and vulnerable a body part is, the more nerve endings it has. The body doesn't distinguish between nerves that signal warning, such as extremes of temperature or pain, from nerves that convey pleasure. In addition to the entire groin area, nerve-rich parts of the body include the ears, the eyelids, the neck, the hands, and the feet.

Aside from the obvious, there aren't usually significant gender differences in which areas of the body feel good (for example, the nipples are usually equally sensitive for men). However, individuals vary greatly. What turns your husband into putty may be a different location than your own preferred hot spots. Find the courage to ask and tell.

Some generally erotic hot zones:

The Lips
Kissing is sorely neglected in most married sex. Kiss often, kiss better, and kiss longer than usual. Try kissing, gently sucking, nibbling, or licking a circle around his lips. Move along from one corner of his

lower lip, across to the other side, then across the upper lip, covering about a half inch of area at a time. Moving very slowly from small area to small area (say, taking two minutes to work your way over both lips) heightens anticipation, ratcheting up the pleasure of the caress as the brain awaits the next sensation.

Great kissing is usually moist but not wet and sloppy. If he gets slobbery, pull back and kiss with dry lips for a bit. Swallow. He'll often unconsciously mimic you. If that doesn't work, tell him that you'd like to try drier kissing. Likewise, go brush your teeth, dragging him along playfully, if he has bad breath.

Assume that all areas of the inside of the mouth are sensitive. Explore his teeth, the inner lips, the roof of his mouth, the crevice just outside the upper and lower gums. Try sucking on just the tip of his tongue as well as rubbing tongues. Add physical contact elsewhere when kissing. Run your hands along his upper arms, place your hand against the back of his neck or lower scalp, or lightly stroke his cheek while kissing. From time to time, open your eyes. Try pulling back a few inches after a few minutes of kissing and really look at each other. Then descend slowly back to his lips with your eyes open.

When moving on to other erotic spots, don't forget to return to kissing. Kissing is often treated as preliminary, something that one does prior to the next sexual step. Try interspersing a few minutes of kissing several times over the course of lovemaking, perhaps even postorgasm. Many men find being kissed after you've been performing oral sex to be highly erotic. Some women enjoy the reverse, while others find the idea of kissing after cunnilingus repugnant.

The Eyes

The eyes are exquisitely sensitive in most individuals. Your partner will naturally close his eyes when you get near, but I'd still advise using your tongue rather than your fingertips to be absolutely sure you don't apply too much pressure. Run your tongue along the base of the eyelashes at the upper lid. Continue in a circular motion just under the eyebrow. Run your tongue along the lower edge of his lashes. Nibble along his eyebrow.

The Ears

Either a massage or oral stimulation of the ear can be very arousing. Try a little oil, warmed in the palm of your hand first, rubbed between your thumb and index finger along the outer edge of the ear. Make a circular motion along the edge, gently pulling down on the earlobes as you finish the movement. Squeeze the upper ear by placing your thumb facing down on the inner aspect, with two or three fingers placed between the upper ear and the scalp line. Pull up gently. This is an acupressure point that releases natural relaxants. The skin just behind the earlobe (at the scalp line) is very sensitive, and some find light massage along the crevice between the back of the ear and the skin is highly erotic.

Ear kissing is heavenly for many, although some people find that the sensation of a tongue placed directly in the entrance to the ear canal to be unpleasant. No one likes wet ear kissing. Blowing directly into the ear is also overrated and sometimes annoying. Tongue-stroking over the areas mentioned above is a better idea. Because the lower earlobe is sensitive but tough, very gently rubbing his lobe between your teeth (and vice versa) can be electrifying.

The Neck

No doubt, you know how wonderfully responsive the neck area is. Pretty much everything feels good here: kissing, nuzzling, light massage. Don't overlook the back of the neck, especially the outer line of muscle that extends from the shoulder into the base of the head. This strategic area is highly nerve-dense. In front, stay away from the center line of the neck, including the Adam's apple and windpipe. The nerve supply here is extremely pressure sensitive, so even mild stimulation can trigger a choking or suffocating sensation.

The Hands

Because of the erotic suggestion of penetration, many partners find that sucking on your fingers or vice versa is very erotic. The webs at the base of each finger are also very sensitive to oral stimulation, as is the center of the palm.

For a great hand massage, grasp your husband's hand by placing your thumb in the center of his palm and your four fingers behind the palm. Rub hand lotion or massage oil into the center of the palm, using your thumb in a firm kneading motion. Adding more lotion as needed, next straighten out your hand, and pull out from the palm along to the tip of his little finger. Repeat for all four fingers, ending with his thumb. Gently encircle each digit as you pull out from the palm. Take a slow count of about five seconds on each finger. Next, intertwine your fingers into his, meeting at the webs. Apply a gentle repeated pressure back and forth at the base of his fingers. Establish a rhythm that is suggestive of the thrusting of intercourse. End by gently kneading the fleshy pads between the bases of the fingers.

The Nipples

In general, men are also very sensitive in their nipples but may be uncomfortable asking for more touch there because it may seem "unmanly." Male nipples respond exactly as female nipples do, so you can gauge your husband's response by noticing the presence and degree of nipple hardening. If his nipples are erect, he likes it. If you've never tried orally stimulating his nipples, you simply must. This is definitely a situation in which what you find pleasurable is likely to be pleasurable for him.

Many men (and women) enjoy a light pressure or pulling of the nipples, perhaps because the hint of painful stimuli is arousing. Again, the best source of feedback is your husband, but to get a general idea of how much pressure to apply in rolling his nipples between your fingertips, take a fold of skin at the back of your left hand between your right thumb and index finger. Rub the skin from side to side between your hands. The level of pressure that doesn't hurt at all is generally the proper amount to apply to his nipples. Instead of merely kissing or licking his nipples, use your mouth to suck in a movement that pulls at the nipple, stretching lightly away from his chest.

Don't neglect, or permit to be neglected, the entire chest/breast area. Capitalize on the pleasure of anticipatory touch by slowly circling your way toward his nipple. Start at about three to five inches away, using very light fingernail pressure. As you reach the nipple, expect that he's likely to prefer the softer touch of your fingertip (or lean in and kiss his nipples at this point). The meridian line down the center of the breastbone is very sensitive in some individuals, so light scratching or nuzzling at the center of the chest may be a particular hot spot.

In general, the penis is the most erotically sensitive area on a man, just as the clitoris is for women. Before you move to caressing his penis, though, take lots of time in the adjacent areas. Keep in mind that as you introduce him to great spots, he's likely to go looking there on your body, so make a convincing argument!

The Feet

If you have ever had a foot massage or pedicure, you don't need to be convinced about how sensitive the feet are. Unfortunately, many of us are inhibited by the vague fear of having a "foot fetish," which somehow has come to symbolize sexual abnormality. There simply is nothing kinky about enjoying the sensuality of a great foot caress.

The bases and webs of the toes, the balls of the feet, and the inner soles are very sensitive to caress (basically, anyplace that is ticklish is potentially erogenous). To avoid triggering a tickle response, make a deeper rubbing motion and/or use lotion or massage oil. If you're comfortable, try licking or sucking between the toes, perhaps after a shared shower.

Inner Thighs

Place your hand behind his knee. Caress in a circular motion over the "knee pit," then slowly run your fingertips or nails along the inner thigh. Spend a lot of time at the crevice between the thigh and the groin. At the crevice, he may appreciate a firmer pressure, which you will know if you 1) ask, or 2) notice that he's pushing into your touch. Before making genital contact, linger at the perineum, one of the most neglected erotic zones that you both will relish.

The Perineum

You may have heard the slang term "taint" for the perineum, so called because "it ain't" the anus and "it ain't" the penis (or vagina). It's the area between the genitals and the anus. In men, the perineum is sometimes called the "male G spot," because it can be as physically exciting as the female "G spot" along the anterior vaginal wall.

(Notice we have both a perineum and a true G spot—no more complaining.)

His perineum is the area from the base of the scrotal sac to the anus. Some men have a distinct "dimple," less than an inch in size, which best corresponds to the "male G spot," although the entire perineal area is highly nerve-rich. When your husband is erect, you may also be able to feel the beginning of the shaft of the penis just adjacent to the scrotal sac. Watch to be sure not to apply too firm a pressure here, especially as you get nearer to the extremely sensitive area of the anus or to the scrotum. If he isn't relaxed because he's worried that you'll scrape or pinch his scrotum, lighten your touch. A light massage here can be intensely pleasurable, although some men greatly enjoy pressure over the perineum, especially over the extension of the penis when erect. If you are turned off by the possibility of touching his anus, or being touched there, relax. There is considerable room to explore before you get to the anus, and the buttocks naturally block off the anus. You have to be trying to find the anus. Stay near the scrotum and you'll be fine. Likewise if he stays just south of your vaginal opening.

The Penis

You already know that your husband's penis is his most erotic zone. You may also know that a common male sexual wish is for more oral sex. If you're uncomfortable with oral sex, it is unlikely that I could say anything that would change your mind. If you're curious but haven't ever tried it, I encourage you to take the leap, because you may really enjoy it. Women who love oral sex describe feeling turned on by the erotic power of giving pleasure as well as the direct visual and tactile feedback of their partner's response.

If you sometimes perform oral sex and are comfortable with it but are either bored by it or have mixed feelings, some things that might make oral sex more enjoyable for you include:

1. Outstanding hygiene. Try getting your point across by performing oral sex during or right after a shower, and say, "I really like how clean you taste."

2. Keep it brief. You don't have to stay there forever, and chances are that he'd prefer a little oral sex more often to the alternative of a lot of oral sex rarely. Make it part of a diverse geographic exploration and stop when *you* want to.

3. Stop before he climaxes. Many women have a strong aversion to ejaculate. Don't think of oral sex as all-or-nothing. If you enjoy giving oral sex but hate for him to climax in your mouth, it's perfectly fine to stop or to ask him to pull away at the moment of climax. It's a compromise he'd probably be happy to make. Don't say, "Oh that stuff really grosses me out." Try instead, "I'd really enjoy more oral sex, and I would like to try it more often if you didn't mind if I stop before you come."

Whether you engage in oral sex or are most comfortable with using your hand to caress his penis, thinking about the subtle geographic differences will make it more exciting for you both. Another way to spice up your touch is to use hypoallergenic lotion, massage oil, or powder, which will greatly change the erotic sensation and add variety. Finally, keep in mind that men generally prefer a more delicate touch at the outset and a firmer one as lovemaking progresses.

Most American men are circumcised. If your husband is not, simply pulling back the foreskin will give you access to the specific areas described here. The single most sensitive spot on the penis is the *frenulum,* the small *Y*-shaped strip of skin that runs from the base of the head of the underside[4] of the penis to the shaft, usually about a quarter inch to a half inch. Some circumcised men have no discernible frenulum, but many have some residual component of this web, which attaches the foreskin to the penis. Touch or graze this area very gently, keeping in mind that it's as nerve-rich as the clitoris.

The next most sensitive part of the penis is the *glans,* which is the head of the penis. The *coronal ridge,* the spot where the glans curves in at the shaft of the penis, is also highly erotic. (The frenulum is located at the midpoint of the coronal ridge, where it faces you during an erection.) Running your tongue around, rotating your fingertips, or forming an *o* with your first finger and thumb and running up and down along the coronal ridge will be well received. Because the underside of the shaft (especially the central line called the *raphe*) and the coronal ridge are more sensitive, many men find it more pleasurable when a woman places her hand "upside down" around the penis, with her thumb on the underside. In other words, your thumb faces his belly button, and your knuckles face you, providing more stimulation from your inner knuckles as your circle up and down along the penis.

The Scrotum

The scrotal sac contains the testicles. Be gentle here but don't avoid this highly erotic area. Try very lightly scratching the skin of the scrotum with your fingernails. Roll each testicle lightly between your fingertips, using no more pressure than you would in handling a raw egg. During penetration, depending on your position, you may be able to reach down and cup one of his testicles or his scrotal sac in

[4]Here and elsewhere, the confusing term "underside" refers to the part of the penis that is closest to the body when the penis is flaccid or soft. During a full erection, this is reversed, and the underside is facing out.

your palm. If you're comfortable doing so, try encircling one of his testicles in your mouth during oral sex.

Female Erotic Geography

Virtually all nongenital geography as described above is equally erotic for women. One of the best reasons to explore new territory or new erotic touches on your husband is that it's a welcome invitation to be explored and touched in the same way. If he doesn't get the point, try something along the lines of "It seems that you really like when I kiss/touch you here/this way. I'd love to see what it feels like when you do that to me."

If You Have Never Climaxed

This book is not about how to have an orgasm if you have not had one before. There are some excellent books on this topic, and I encourage you to make this a priority if you haven't had an orgasm before. If you aren't sure whether you're having orgasms, you're not. I can tell you this: It all boils down to finding the right touch in the right spot.

Every book you find on becoming orgasmic will tell you what you may not wish to hear: You almost certainly will need to self-explore through masturbation. You need to find the right spot before you can help him find it.

The other surefire way is to experiment with a vibrator. It's virtually a guarantee that you can bring yourself to climax if you're willing to use a vibrator (more about considering sex "toys" in Step Nine). There is also a new medical device that enhances the likelihood of orgasm, called the Eros-Therapy (described in Step Ten).

The Right Spot: The Clitoris

The statistics in the next box illustrate an important geographical lesson: the clitoris is *the* key spot for orgasm. The clitoris is the only human organ whose sole purpose is sexual pleasure. The clitoris has as many nerve cells as the entire penis, but all in one concentrated location. Unfortunately, intercourse is a pretty indirect route to the clitoris, and I want you to fully appreciate that geographically, vaginal intercourse is not the road to greater sexual pleasure for most women.

- Fewer than 1 in 3 women always have an orgasm with a partner.
- Only 20 percent to 30 percent of women ever climax during coitus alone (most regularly orgasmic women climax during oral or manual stimulation).
- Eight percent to ten percent of women rarely or never climax. One in four married women have an orgasm "sometimes" or never.
- Many women are situationally orgasmic, meaning that they can climax during certain sexual acts, such as receiving oral sex or masturbating, but not during others, including vaginal intercourse.
- You are more likely to always orgasm if you are African American or Hispanic, religiously conservative, or did not graduate from college. However, these factors are trivial compared with the fact that the single highest predictor of regular orgasm is being male.

This is one reason why the concept of "foreplay" is so insensitive to women's bodies: foreplay for whom? It suggests that the very activities most likely to lead to orgasm in women don't count as much as the "real play" of intercourse. A major reason why some women find sex boring is because they're stuck thinking vaginal intercourse is supposed to be the peak experience. Trying to climax during intercourse can be frustrating or seem like an indictment of your sexual inferiority.

If you're looking to increase pleasure, start with the clitoris. If you've already discovered that, stop blaming yourself for the fact that your body was designed with this incredibly sensitive spot located *outside* the vagina. Some women who don't always climax would do so if intercourse lasted longer, which would result in longer indirect stimulation of the clitoris. Sex researchers and pioneers Masters and Johnson proved without a doubt that the average woman takes approximately three times as long to reach climax as her male partner. If her partner could postpone his own climax, some women would be more likely to climax during intercourse.

If you're raising children in the twenty-first century, you came of sexual age when Freud's claim that clitorally-based orgasm was inferior to vaginally-based orgasm had already been debunked (by Masters and Johnson in the 1960s). Unfortunately, many moms also became sexually active before the G spot, named after a German physician named Grafenberg, was understood. Indeed, even now, not all researchers agree that there is such a thing as a G spot. One area of controversy is whether G-spot orgasms differ from clitoral orgasms. Let's get away from the emphasis on orgasm potency (is there a bad orgasm?), and consider the G spot as a source of enhanced sexual pleasure, uncontroversially a good thing.

Currently, we believe that the G spot may actually be an extension of the clitoris, which is a partially vaginally embedded organ composed of erectile tissue and much larger than was previously recognized. What we think of as the clitoris is actually the glans, or head, of the clitoris. That nub of tissue we've called the clitoris is as much the whole clitoris as the glans or head of the penis is the whole penis.[5] You may already have discovered your G spot. If you notice that a certain position of intercourse results in the head of your partner's penis pressing on a particularly erogenous spot in the upper vaginal wall, that's it. Or if you have noticed that during oral or manual stimulation of your external genitalia, when your partner inserts a finger in your vagina and pushes upward toward your belly, you feel a noticeably enhanced pleasure, then he is contacting your G spot. Some women climax during oral sex much more readily or more powerfully with G spot pressure. Try it by guiding your husband's finger into your vagina during oral sex.

If you aren't sure where the G spot is, you probably haven't found it. You can locate it yourself, or ask your partner to go on a G-spot exploration with you. To find it yourself, first empty your bladder. While sitting on the toilet, insert your index finger in your vagina, aiming centrally on the upper, or front, wall of the vagina, approximately a half finger's depth. Move your fingertip around until you locate a spongy, pea- or dime-sized area that is especially sensitive: You're there. During lovemaking, this area is much more sensitive and is an especially good spot for your husband to massage.

Because the clitoris extends above (toward the belly button) the glans as well as along the sides and into the vaginal opening, you may find that your partner's extra attention to the surrounding area is highly stimulating. In fact, Drs. Marcia and Lisa Douglass coined the term "cligeva,"[6] an amalgam of "clitoris–G spot–vagina." Most

[5]For more about male and female anatomy and physiology, I recommend Drs. Jennifer and Laura Berman, *For Women Only* (New York: Henry Holt and Company, 2001).

[6]Marcia Douglass and Lisa Douglass, *Are We Having Fun Yet? The Intelligent Woman's Guide to Sex* (New York: Hyperion, 1997).

women find that the clitoris is the most pleasurable location, followed by the G spot, followed by the vagina. It makes sense to conceptualize the geography as one continuous erotic zone, not that different from the penis in having differentially sensitive areas.

Some women find that the area surrounding the urethra, the opening of the tube that drains the bladder, is also very erotic. Some find that tapping the cervix, either by finger or by deep vaginal penetration during intercourse, is also exquisitely pleasurable. Others, however, find one or both of these spots to be uncomfortable.

Finally, as mentioned before, one in five women have tried anal intercourse. People aren't usually in the middle about anal touching or intercourse. Either you think it's distasteful or you are curious and perhaps already include it in your sexuality. The anus is very rich in sensory nerve supply and some perfectly nice moms really like to be touched there. Some find it geographically as pleasing as the clitoris, given the intensity of the sensory supply and the pleasure of disregarding taboo. If you'd like to explore this, I recommend *The Ultimate Guide to Anal Sex for Women,* by Tristan Taormino (Cleiss Press, 1997).

Go for the Whirlwind Tour of the Tourist Attractions

As you explore new geography, please also remember to break the rules about timing. You know the rules of your relationship: first this, then this, then that, then we're done. Reject the concept of "foreplay" in every possible way, including the idea of what comes when. There is no set order in which to make love. Interrupt your touches and go back to kissing. Interrupt penetration to go back to caressing one another. Move from the back of his neck to his inner thigh to his toes and back to kissing. Mix it up!

Erotic Anatomy and Intercourse

For most women, there are certain positions for intercourse that are more pleasurable. Of course, some of how you prefer to be in contact is not at all about pelvic anatomy, but may be more reflective of how much skin-to-skin contact you enjoy, how your or his back feels, whether you feel self-conscious in a particular position, how eye contact enhances the experience for you, or how you feel emotionally about positions that suggest aggression and/or passivity.

I imagine that most readers have experimented, and many have already discovered what is most pleasurable for them. While most couples make love in only a few different positions, you may have fallen into a missionary habit that is worth breaking. Another potential bad habit is relinquishing control of decision making to your husband. If he enjoys a position that you hate, speak up. If you enjoy a position that he never initiates, take charge.

The possibilities are endless, and I want to assure you that there isn't the equivalent of a secret handshake that you don't know. A few tips that might be useful:

Missionary position (total frontal contact, man on top). Tilting your pelvis up may increase stimulation to the G spot. The easiest way to do this is to put one or two pillows under your bottom. This classic position will be even more pleasurable for you both if you tighten your buttocks and pelvic floor (remember those Kegel exercises from childbirth preparation class?). Also try removing the pillow from under your head so that your upper body is flat against the mattress. A comfortable, interesting variation for many is facing each other while lying on your sides (your legs will be interwoven).

Woman on top (reverse missionary with your knees bent and supporting your weight). Women who enjoy cervical contact may like this position especially. It also provides perfect access for either your partner or yourself to simultaneously massage your clitoris and may increase the likelihood of a female coital orgasm. (I know that some readers are gasping at the notion of self-stimulation during intercourse. It may help to know that men report that watching their partner masturbate is an extremely common and powerful fantasy.) Some women are too self-conscious about stomach flab to enjoy being on top. He's not noticing.

Modified missionary position (also called coital alignment). When your husband penetrates, your natural response is to open your legs and knees, placing his legs in between your own. Try this variation: Once he penetrates, straighten your legs under him, crossing at your ankles. His legs will naturally end up outside and along your own. This position pulls the penis into a great anatomical alignment with the clitoris and G spot. To maximize penile-clitoral contact, he should move his pelvis slightly forward after penetration (called "pelvic override") and rock back and forth. The base of the penis should rub against your clitoris. Okay, I lied. *This* is the secret handshake—try it!

Spoon (female faces forward, male behind her also facing forward). You can do this side by side with each of you contacting the bed at the hip and shoulder, or with the female on her hands and knees while he grasps her hips or lower back. Placing several pillows under your abdomen and chest may make this more comfortable for you. He enters the vagina from the rear, which some women find gives deeper penetration, allowing for better cervical contact. It also gives much better access to the clitoris during penetration than missionary intercourse. Some women find the position Shakespeare described as "the beast with two backs" unappealing, either because it feels less intimate without face-to-face contact or because it seems uncivilized. Don't engage in positions or types of intercourse that make you uncomfortable.

Get Complicated

Simply surprising your partner by switching positions midstream instantly makes sex more interesting. The subtle changes in how your bodies make contact awakens the sensory brain, and something you've done a hundred times before is suddenly more sensual. Men also appreciate women taking the lead in switching positions because it telegraphs interest and enthusiasm. If you're uncomfortable using words, body language is a direct and effective way to make your point. And anything that communicates engagement is erotic.

Savor All That Is Erotic

When we are too young to know our bodies, too young to speak our minds, too young to take risks in our relationships, we're blessed with such great chemistry that we don't even notice that we're making love in the rushed and rather blundering manner of youth. Sure, the fiery passion of tearing off your clothes the second you got inside the door was great, and, no, that's not coming back. But the good news is that the best sex is sex with someone you trust. We are perfectly biologically designed for a lifetime of sexual pleasure, if we find the courage to be vulnerable.

You *can* have more adventurous sex with a trusted spouse.

Increasing novelty in lovemaking, like becoming more mindful in the bedroom, is a process rather than a destination. It's a lifelong approach that can be adapted to the ebbs and flows of any sexual relationship, be they the birth of another child, the natural changes of aging, periods of serious illnesses, or even entertaining houseguests. It takes practice, but it quickly becomes second nature.

The fundamental change requires mentally cleansing the notion that the pinnacle of lovemaking is when a penis enters a vagina. A commitment to invigorating sexuality requires attention to the erotic potential of the entire body, and the conscious decision to accentuate the physical senses. It's profoundly natural in the best sense of the term. We are graced with complex, rich sensory receptors and bodies that offer us endlessly interesting possibilities.

Affirmation
"Live out of your imagination, not your history."
—Stephen Covey

Phase Three
ACCEPT the WISDOM of OTHERS

So far, we've looked at developing and strengthening the resources you already have within your sexual relationship. The final steps to great sex involve exploring the world outside for new and helpful ways to reclaim passion.

Great sex does not depend on endless variation or toys. You can have great sexual intimacy with the resources and products in this section, and you can have great sexual intimacy without them. Great sex is characterized by love, trust, spiritual connection, vulnerability, attentiveness, enthusiasm, mutuality, and respect. Batteries are optional. Some readers need permission to explore, others need specific advice about taking advantage of the marketplace.

In Step Eight, I will suggest that you borrow from those women willing to share their sexy imaginations with you. There are writers, editors, and filmmakers who have created stories, novels, books, and videos that you can enjoy in the privacy of your bedroom.

I'll also tell you about the entrepreneurs who want to make your shopping experience (for these and other sensual products) as pleasant as a trip to the finest department store.

Within these steps, I will make specific suggestions for the mild to the downright racy. Pick and choose according to what is comfortable within your own relationship. This is far from exhaustive, so if you find a particular approach that really revs your engine, you'll have a good starting place.

Borrowing and buying from other women is a tradition as old as time.

Stay open to possibility. Keep an open mind. You are free to reject any of these ideas, but try to consider all possibilities before deciding what may suit you.

Step Eight: Borrow Your Way to Great Sex

> "Many couples . . . want to broaden their sexual horizons as a way to further enhance their intimacy, much as you might add new flowers to the garden—not because you have tired of the old, but because you desire something different."
>
> —Lonnie Garfield Barbach, Ph.D., *The Erotic Edge: Erotica for Couples*

- Actively using sexual fantasy to enliven your sexual experience is an option. There are many ways to borrow other women's erotic imaginations.
- Woman-centered, woman-created erotica can be free of the domination, sexual violence, ethnic stereotyping, and interpersonal exploitation that we associate with pornography. There is a genre of fiction that is female friendly, thoughtful, sensual, dignified, and mature.
- The Web and online bookstores permit you access to erotic material in privacy.

This chapter is not for every reader. I invite you to skip this if you are absolutely, unconditionally certain that you would not consider anything along the lines of an erotic book or conscious use of fantasy to boost your libido.

But . . . if there is a sliver of possibility that you might be intrigued by some new approaches, read on. There is a universe created by your sisters that you can borrow to add spice to your bedroom.

I promised no black leather Swedish dominatrix costumes, and I mean it. "Way too kinky" is, of course, in the eye of the beholder. I'm pretty certain, however, that none of the suggestions in this chapter challenges my credentials as a feminist, a physician, or a real mom. I also hope that my own mother and my own children never read these next two chapters. This is an intensely private and sensitive topic, best restricted to a committed sexual relationship or your own head.

Anything new is uncomfortable at the beginning, and sexual exploration is an especially vulnerable endeavor. We fear feeling or seeming foolish. Expect to feel a little foolish or clumsy. It's okay. Stop or avoid things that feel ludicrous or more weird than exciting. Read this chapter with the knowledge that you have permission to explore, but there are no obligations.

Even if you feel quite comfortable trying new things, you may need information and guidance. Women in our culture—especially mothers—are explicitly and implicitly discouraged from useful sexual discourse. For example, one study found that fewer than one in five postpartum women was advised by her obstetrician about sexual changes or problems after childbirth at her six-week checkup. How striking. Even the population of known sexually active mothers is neglected by physicians who specialize in vaginas! You also won't find much practical information on sexuality in the parenting section of the bookstore, and you won't find anything on mothers in the sexuality section.

You may find searching for woman-friendly erotic materials annoying or embarrassing. You may have to weed through Web pages filled with offensive photographs, nervously leaf through the highly variable offerings at the local bookstore, or find that the online store that claims to market to the timid seems outrageous to you.

The song says sisters are doing it for themselves, and this has certainly been the case over the last ten years of women's erotic material. Women writers, women filmmakers, and women entrepreneurs have quietly revolutionized the field. We have choices, products, and literature that speaks to us, but we have to know where to find it.

Remember, the Banner Labeled "Normal" Is Wide

In choosing descriptions of the categories, I'm aware of the risk of labeling certain ideas "tame" and others "wild." Each reader will have a comfort zone that is uniquely hers. If you read this chapter and don't find a single idea you'd consider actually doing, please don't conclude that you're frigid or repressed. If you read this chapter and don't find a single idea you haven't already tried or considered, please don't conclude that you're a sexual daredevil. The goal is to nurture your own intrinsic sexual imagination and creativity, but only to the point at which it feels integrated and authentic to you. I include labels to give you permission and possibility. I also hope that if you have explored some of these ideas but feel sheepish, you'll make peace with your sexual curiosity.

Sexual Fantasy

All human beings do or can fantasize sexually. If you have absolutely no fantasies at all, you may have a chemical problem caused by testosterone deficiency or antidepressant medication, or you may be struggling to overcome a Puritanical upbringing that told you that fantasizing is shameful.

More commonly, we've ignored or let our sexual fantasies wither, perhaps because we have spent every spare iota of energy on our kids. Yet sexual fantasies are normal, healthy, and energizing. Adding more fantasy before or during lovemaking is highly time efficient for parents and an easy way to invigorate boring sex.

It isn't true that "anything goes." Not all fantasizing is perfectly fine, and you don't have to agree to explore problematic fantasies just because your partner says you should. Fantasies that are problematic include sexual disorders (forced sex, pedophilia, incest) or anything that makes you uncomfortable. Some fantasies could be hurtful if shared. No one wants to hear that her partner is fantasizing about someone else, even if she's doing it, too. Finally, one can have too much of a good thing, when fantasy excludes the here-and-now, creates distance, or diminishes mindfulness.

Try using fantasy in two ways. First, deliberately call up fantasies from time to time when you aren't making love. This is especially useful for women who rarely initiate sex or whose libido generally lags behind their husbands'. Many women know exactly when he is likely to initiate sex (e.g., it's Saturday night) but find it difficult to warm up to the idea of lovemaking in advance. If this is you, you're the perfect candidate for consciously fantasizing for a few moments throughout the day. Sure, you may never spontaneously think about sex. But you certainly have the choice to override a sleepy libido by *deciding* to think sexually.

Second, fantasize while making love, sometimes. Like anything sexual, avoid repetition or overreliance on fantasy as a way to become aroused. Keep it fresh. You might want to imagine your husband doing your very favorite thing while he's actually doing something not so interesting. Or you might try one or more of the following three gradations of spiciness.

Starting with the mild: Try fantasizing about making love with your husband in a *different place.* Common sexual fantasies you can borrow include making love:

- outdoors (at the beach, in a park, in the woods);
- in your own or a fantasy house (in front of the fireplace, on the table, on the kitchen floor, against a door);
- in a watery spot (a hot tub, swimming pool, in the shower);
- in a totally inappropriate site (your office, his office, a department store, between the church pews);
- in a potentially risky/public place (an elevator, a hotel balcony, an airplane, a movie theater).

Moving up on the fantasy scale, imagine making love with *someone else*. Many readers already do this, most probably feeling very guilty about it. Fantasy is make-believe. It doesn't mean that you are about to have an affair or wish you weren't making love to your partner.

Common alternative sexual partner fantasies you can borrow include:

- former lovers;
- men in uniform (policemen, military, firemen);
- workmen;
- one's boss, a coworker, or an employee;
- doctors;
- clergymen (yes, being forbidden is sexy for many);
- television or movie actors;
- singers, musicians, or other celebrities;
- an extremely slow, sensual, lingering, and patient lover whose sole goal is to give you sexual pleasure.

At the spiciest end of the scale are fantasies that are often not possible or not something you would do, generally in the category of things you wouldn't tell your shrink about. These are the fantasies that worry us or make us feel "weird." But these are extremely common female sexual fantasies and not pathological. Don't be alarmed if you enjoy fantasizing about *things you might not or even never would actually do.* You may wish to borrow some of the following:

- sex with a stranger;
- being watched while making love or watching others make love;
- sex with more than one partner (either another man, or a woman);
- making love with whipped cream, chocolate sauce, or other food;
- dominating the sexual encounter;
- willingly submitting to a sexual encounter;
- teaching an inexperienced twenty-something how to make love;
- sex in a historical romance (on a pirate ship, in the Old West, as a nurse tending to wounded soldiers).

There are books devoted to this topic. I recommend *Private Thoughts: Exploring the Power of Women's Sexual Fantasies,* by Wendy Maltz and Suzie Boss (New World Library, 2001). If you've never ordered a book online, this might be one to start with. The additional cost of postage is usually offset by a discount off the cover price, and it's a private transaction. The mail carrier doesn't have a clue what's in there, and your nanny won't guess either. One of the great features of online book shopping is that the major sites offer suggestions for related books. If you find a book you like, it's very easy to find similar items. (A word of caution: amazon.com suggests similar books to those you've previously purchased at subsequent sign-in screens. This could be a problem if you're logging on with your kid standing next to you looking for the latest Animorphs book.)

Author Nancy Friday has written several compilations of women's sexual fantasies, breaking the taboo barrier in 1973 with *My Secret*

[1]See Laframboise's Web site, www.razberry.com/pink/top.htm.

Garden: Women's Sexual Fantasies (Pocket, 1998). Some readers adore her works; others find her anything-goes approach a bit over the top. Before you buy, go to www.barnesandnoble.com and read the sample chapter online.

Incorporating Fantasy into Lovemaking

If you have a creative bent when it comes to sexual fantasies, you can tell each other erotic fantasies while making love. Take a fantasy, such as making love in the woods, and tell him a story. If you have trouble starting, practice setting the stage in your head one time, then share the details next time. Begin with a romantic place you've been together, and start with "Remember when we were walking on that beach in California. I'm imagining that we're there alone in the moonlight, walking hand in hand on the sand. No one is around, and you . . ." You can get very explicit or stay very vague. It's the intentionality and the excitement of telling a story while making love that makes this so hot.

Erotic Literature

If you've ever read a romance novel, face it: You've read erotic literature. You've borrowed someone else's erotic fantasies in the form of a novel. Women spend nearly a billion dollars a year on romance novels, and, as journalist Donna Laframboise notes, "Romance novels are many women's version of *Penthouse.* . . . the point isn't that all women respond to such stimuli, but that some do. Anyone who believes in female self-determination must acknowledge and respect this fact."

Romance novels run the gamut from delicate "we were fated to be together" love stories (such as those by Nora Roberts or Judith McNaught) to kidnapping by rich and handsome warriors who go on to marry the heroines whose virginity they've stolen (à la Johanna Lindsey and Heather Graham). They all include sensuality and textual erotica. If you find that you are aroused by romance novels, let go of any self-consciousness and enjoy the fantasies. If you've never picked one up, give it a try. Take charge, perhaps retiring to your bedroom to get your fire going while your husband puts the kids to bed. Don't expect anything approaching reality: Romance novel orgasms are simultaneous, multiple, coital, and generally have little to do with what actually happens in real women's bedrooms.

Some women find romance novels to be silly, embarrassing, implausible, or highly repetitive and predictable. These readers may enjoy sexy literature. Some very sexy literary novels include Terry McMillan's *How Stella Got Her Groove Back* (Signet, 1998), Laura Esquivel's *Like Water for Chocolate* (Anchor, 1994), Alison Lurie's *Foreign Affairs* (the 1985 Pulitzer Prize winner; reissued by Avon, 1995), Alice Hoffman's *Practical Magic* (Berkley, 1995), Jeanette Winterson's *Written on the Body* (Vintage, 1994), and Linda Jaivin's *Eat Me* (Broadway, 1997). Two very sexy novels written by men are Milan Kundera's *The Unbearable Lightness of Being* (Harper, 1999) and Nicholson Baker's *Vox: A Novel* (Vintage, 1995).

Sexy literary fiction has some great advantages over women's erotica. You can read it on the beach or the train without worrying about creeps following you. You can buy it when you're with the kids. You can feed your brain as well as your sexual mind. It's generally tamer and so more appealing for some women. But it's not time efficient. Erotica is quick and to the point, more like shots of tequila than sherry. Explicitly erotic fiction is there for those seeking a quick jolt.

If you haven't looked into women's erotica in the last ten years, you're in for a very pleasant surprise. It isn't what you think. Things are really different than the days of *The Story of O,* when female authorship didn't make any difference in content: It was still about humiliation, sexual slavery, rape, and abuse. Women have now claimed the field as insiders, infusing the genre with what Simone de Beauvoir predicted would be "a special form of (our) own . . . a sensuality, a sensitivity, of a special nature."[1]

Woman-centered erotica is, by definition, "softer," less phallic-centered, and far more likely to involve caring relationships. Of course, women may create and enjoy a wide variety of sexual themes, and I don't want to leave you with the idea that women's erotica is fundamentally dainty. The collections I'll describe below range from mild to wild; some of it is exceptionally well written, some not. Many wonderful collections appeal to women of either a lesbian or a heterosexual orientation, while others are primarily heterosexually oriented. It's a myth that women's erotica is just for lesbians, although most erotica collections are inclusive in terms of sexual orientation. Some appeal to your baddest bad girl fantasies, while others speak to the mildly naughty. Published works of erotica are usually short stories, and as for all collected works, you'll like some and not others.

In addition to finding the voice that speaks to your sexuality, you will need to figure out how to incorporate erotic literature into your relationship. The Web has numerous collections of women's erotic literature, and you can explore this privately to cultivate your sexual mind. Your husband doesn't need to know what you did during the baby's nap. Or you might be perfectly comfortable if your husband knows that you've decided to explore this option. You might even consider reading erotic poems or stories to one another as part of lovemaking.

[1]Simone de Beauvoir, *The Second Sex* (1949), translated by H. M. Parshley (New York: Bantam, 1970).

Privacy is an important issue for mothers, but an obstacle that can be easily overcome. Keep your literature locked away from the kids. As mentioned, you get complete privacy when you purchase books online.[2] The three major online bookstores, amazon.com, barnes-andnoble.com, or borders.com, all sell women's erotic fiction. Enter "women's erotica" in any of their search engines or look for the following selections:

Choices for the Mildly Curious

Touching Fire: Erotic Writings by Women, edited by Laura Thornton, Jan Sturtevant, and Amber Coverdale Sumrall. (New York: Carroll & Graf, 1989). This book is one of the pioneering works in mainstream published women's erotica. Almost equally divided between prose and poetry, the literary quality is outstanding (contributors include Zora Neale Hurston, Marge Piercy, Adrienne Rich, and Margaret Atwood). The writings are gentle, sensitive, pleasingly multicultural, and mother-friendly. Don't miss Cathryn Alpert's "Where We Are Now," because you just have to love erotica that features forty-four-year-old parents making love in a car littered with Gummi Bear wrappers. Sharon Olds' poetic ode to the postpartum healing power of oral sex ("New Mother") also shouldn't be missed.

The Penguin Book of Erotic Stories by Women, edited by Richard Glyn Jones and A. Susan Williams (New York: Penguin, 1996). This is a somewhat awkwardly compiled assortment of erotica, whose main point seems to be that highly respected authors have written erotica. There is a little bit of everything, including science fiction, world literature, stilted prose, gorgeous writing, gentle romance,

[2]In addition to privacy, the online bookstores often include reader comments, which will help you get a feel for whether a book might appeal to you.

and the downright kinky. Some of the better entries include "Violette" (how you only wish you'd lost your virginity), Isabel Allende's "Our Secret," and Ann Oakley's "Where the Bee Sucks."

Choices for the More Adventurous

Some erotica appeals to readers of all sexual orientations and the wide range of human sexual fantasies. If you're ready to really take the plunge, and keep that internal censor knob turned way down, you won't go wrong with any of the following:

The Best American Erotica 2001, edited by Susie Bright (New York: Touchstone Books, 2001). This collection of erotic short stories also includes a great directory of Web sites and publishers. Highly readable. The series originated as the *Herotica* series (1992 through 1999). Volumes 1 through 3 are edited by the grande dame of women's erotica, Susie Bright, and volumes 4 through 6 are edited by noted erotica writer Marcie Sheiner. Choose any. In fact, you won't go wrong with any of the numerous collections edited by either Bright or Sheiner, whose anthologies include a mix of unknown and famous authors. For excerpts from the *Best American Erotica* and the *Herotica* series, see www.susiebright.com.

The Erotic Edge: Erotica for Couples, edited by Lonnie Garfield Barbach (New York: Plume, 1996). Approximately half the stories are written by women, although all are intended to be of interest to couples (not necessarily heterosexual). Highly readable.

Aqua Erotica: 18 Stories for a Steamy Bath, edited by Mary Anne Mohanraj (New York: Three Rivers Press, 2000). This cleverly conceived book is waterproof, and all stories include water themes. About half of the entries are by women (including noted writer Louise Erdrich), with plenty of mermaids, hot tubs, and beaches. Try reading stories out loud during a shared erotic bath.

There are three specialty collections of women's erotica of note:

Best Black Women's Erotica, edited by Blanche Richardson (San Francisco: Cleis Press, 2000).

The Oy of Sex: Jewish Women Write Erotica, edited by Marcy Sheiner (San Francisco: Cleis Press, 1999).

Zaftig: Well Rounded Erotica, edited by Hanne Blank (San Francisco: Cleis Press, 2001), body-positive erotica for large women.

Erotica on the Web

There is almost a limitless amount of erotica on the Web. Reading erotica on the Web has certain advantages: it's free, private, requires no secret storage spot, and ranges from mild to exceptionally wild. You can find erotic poetry, fiction, photography, drawings, and video clips.

The disadvantages are significant, however. First, there is no editor—you weed through it yourself. Secondly, many erotica sites have commercial pop-up banners that are deeply offensive and intended to appeal to teenage boys. However, the Web may be a place to discover whether erotic literature appeals to you before committing to building a library.

If you wish to peruse the Web privately, unless you clear the Internet history file, any subsequent users, including your technology-savvy teenager, can see which sites you've visited. Many Internet servers use Microsoft Internet Explorer. To clear the history file, begin at a neutral Web address (i.e., leave the erotic site and go to something bland like www.allrecipes.com). Next, go to the "View" button at the top of the toolbar. Click "View," which will open a scroll-down list. Click "Internet Options," usually at the bottom of the menu. You will see three icons, including "History." At the right of the History icon, you will see the button "Clear history." When you click this, you will be asked "Delete all items in your history folder?" Confirm by clicking "yes," which will delete only previous Web addresses visited (and won't affect your saved "favorites" folder).

On AOL 6.0, click on "Settings" on the toolbar. Go to "Preferences" and select "Toolbar" from the left column of choices. Click on "Clear history now." To confirm that you've successfully cleared the history on any Internet service, try to click the drop-down arrow to the right of the address bar. There should be no Web addresses beneath the page you are currently visiting. If you're having trouble clearing the Web address bar, go to help on your server, and search for "clear history."

In addition to clearing your internet history folder, you will want to make sure visiting erotic sites on the web doesn't trigger a flurry of unwanted e-mail offers for sexual products. If you end up on such a list, you may get e-mail with subject lines that would make you cringe were you to open your mailbox with someone looking over your shoulder. Most computers accept what are termed cookies (a file that opens the door to further e-mail offers as well as stores passwords) unless specifically told not to by the user.

To avoid getting cookies while browsing for erotic literature or products using:

Internet Explorer 6.0: Click Tools. Click Internet Options. Choose the Privacy tab. Select high.

Internet Explorer 5.x (5.1, 5.2 etc.): Click Tools. Click Internet Options. Choose the Security tab. Select high.

AOL: Click Settings. Click Preferences. Click Internet Properties. Choose the Security tab. Select High.

You will probably wish to lower the security settings back to your default level (usually medium or medium high) so that you can use the web more efficiently during nonerotic visits.

Don't even *think* about checking out these Web sites on your office computer.

A few sites that include anything-goes erotic fiction without excessive triple-X pop-up advertisements include:

www.cleansheets.com
www.scarletletters.com
www.erotica-readers.com
www.nerve.com

One way to access erotic writing without the intrusive commercials for porn sites is to explore sexuality sites that offer commentary, advice, and/or what-I-once did memoirs. I recommend the following:

http://www.salon.com/sex/index.html. I can't say enough good things about this site. While you're at salon.com, search for archived Susie Bright columns and check out the sometimes sexual "Mothers Who Think" features.

http://www.hipmama.com. Click on the "hip talk" icon, then scroll down to the "sex" bulletin board.

http://www.goaskalice.columbia.edu/Cat6.html. Columbia University health advice, mostly targeted at college students, but you'll find some interesting ideas here.

You might enjoy reading bulletin board postings made by visitors to women's Web sites such as www.oxygen.com or www.ivillage.com. Understand that while these bulletin board sites are unedited and often meandering, you might like reading the erotic musings of real women. You might also get an erotic charge by posting your questions or stories.

If you discover a passion for the Web and would like to explore all that it has to offer in the way of erotic material, you can find hundreds of sites in Anne Seman and Cathy Winks' *The Woman's Guide to Sex on the Web* (HarperSanFrancisco, 1999).

Go Ahead—Take It!

Borrowing erotic fantasies and fiction for use in your own bedroom is exactly what these writers have in mind! Bedtime stories for grown-ups exist because there's a market, a *huge* market. As Susie Bright points out, erotica for women "must be the fastest-growing fiction genre ever seen."[3] The market for well-written, sensitive, woman-positive erotic literature exploded over the last ten years because creative and sexually empowered women discovered the need and a desire for it. This is an easy, side-effect-free, private, low-cost, no-calorie way to great sex. You can use it alone, or you can include it in lovemaking. Whatever you decide works best for you, give it a try before deciding it won't work at all.

Affirmation
"A person will be called to account on Judgment Day for every permissible thing he might have enjoyed but did not."
—The Talmud

[3]Susie Bright, ed., *The Best American Erotica 2001* (New York: Touchstone Books, 2001), p. 7.

Step Nine: Shop Your Way to Great Sex

"... self-empowerment has been partially responsible for bringing sex toys out of the velvety shadows of porn shops and into a new arena of sexual health and pleasure."

—Annie Auguste, "This Toy Is Not a Toy," *www.salon.com*

- You may find that your sexual intimacy is enriched by actively exploring erotic films targeted to women.
- You can also play together in ways that add spice to your intimacy.
- Some women will find that a vibrator is a great option that can greatly enhance sexual pleasure.

In Step One, I asked you to start throwing spare change into a jar at the end of the day. Now we're going to start spending your money.

Visually Erotic Material

It is often noted that visual stimuli are especially arousing for men, an observation supported by market for nude magazines and porn films. In contrast, women are more sensitive to tactile and auditory stimuli. Some women do enjoy sexually explicit visual imagery, while many do not, or do not enjoy traditional "adult entertainment," such as the type of video rentals found in hotels.

However, most of us do like a good "romantic" movie, and it's perfectly okay to decide to watch a sexy movie to increase your libido. Deciding to watch a steamy video for the sole purpose of getting ready to make love later in the evening is erotic and different than dragging your reluctant husband to a chick flick. Some videos you might want to watch in order to increase your lust include *Bull Durham, The English Patient, Like Water for Chocolate,* and *Shakespeare in Love.* To take it up a notch, try renting *9 1/2 Weeks, The Kama Sutra,* or a French-subtitled, sexy romance (all available at ordinary video rental stores).

There is also a new body of X-rated films specifically marketed to women. These are visually explicit, sexual (even the ones described as having a strong plot are sex flicks), and created for the sole purpose of sexual pleasure. Unlike women's erotica, where the difference is partly literary, the difference in woman-positive erotic films has more to do with an absence of fake-breasted cheerleaders than it does with artistic value.

Women who have in the past reluctantly watched an adult film with their husbands may find women-centered erotic films to be a far more appealing alternative. Again, no one should do anything they don't enjoy in the bedroom solely to please a partner, but consider trying something once.

Whether you want to sample a traditional hotel-porn video (which will cost you around $10), rent a sexy R-rated video from Blockbuster ($4), or purchase a women-positive sex flick, you can use these films in the same way you use erotica: alone or with your partner. Watching a sexy film alone in anticipation of lovemaking, behind a locked door while your husband puts the kids to bed, is a great way to persuade him of the merits of putting the kids to bed. It's win-win.

We know why hotels have videos: for men to view during masturbation. That's an option for you, too. More sex leads to more sex, and self-knowledge leads to better sex. You might find that masturbating while watching a sexy film increases your comfort with your body and raises your general sexiness quotient, which translates into better couple sex.

But women tend to use erotic films differently than men. We're more comfortable using them as part of lovemaking. The challenge for parents is finding the appropriate opportunity. An erotic film is just about the last thing you want your kids hearing or discovering you enjoying. This tends to require planning, although one of the advantages of owning your own video is that you can lock it away and grab it when the opportunity arises.

Some alternatives: an overnight at a bed-and-breakfast that has an in-room VCR, a lunch date while the kids are at school, an unexpected free evening when the kids all happen to get invited out for sleepovers, right after you drop your child off at a birthday party, or, for the truly wicked, when Grandma takes them to church or synagogue.

Why are films erotic for some women? Part of it appeals to the voyeur. Many sexual fantasies and erotic writings capture the forbidden but erotic pleasure of being a sexual observer. Part of it is just that it's naughty, which is sexy all by itself. Also, while women are less likely to be visually triggered to want sex, auditory input is a stronger trigger for women, and leaving the film running in the background enhances the erotic experience for some women.

I believe that part of what's sexy for couples is that it takes trust and vulnerability to do something so racy together. It's being a couple that makes it especially sensual to share the experience, which is what distinguishes making love from mating.

If I've convinced you to give it a try, start with a video made by filmmaker Candida Royalle, whose Femme Productions is specifically dedicated to "give adult movies a woman's voice and explore what we women desire." As an example, Royalle's critically acclaimed *Christine's Secret* is sexually egalitarian: Woman climax as often as men and receive as much oral sex as they give. They also laugh and cuddle postcoitally, and one sex scene features a long-married yet passionate couple.

Royalle's videos (and even a DVD, a highly efficient way to return to favorite scenes) are available (generally at a better price than elsewhere) at her Web site, www.royalle.com.html or by phone at 1-800-456-5683. Many of her films are also available at the Good Vibrations site (see below).

An entirely different approach is that of filmmaker Veronica Hart, who makes what she terms "ultraexplicit" sex films. Her *Love's Passion* is a best-seller at Good Vibes. The story line involves a romance novelist's imagined Civil War–era sexual reunion, interspersed with the current escapades of her friends. In addition to a romance-based theme, the paid escort in this film is male, the men don't balk at condoms, and the women love sex, which is never nonconsensual. Otherwise, the film has much in common with male-produced porn. The visuals are so explicit that they're almost gynecologic, and some viewers will be turned off by the threesomes, anal sex, and augmented breasts. Others will be turned on.

You can find this and other Veronica Hart films at the woman-owned Web site Good Vibrations (www.goodvibes.com), which has an extensive collection of erotic videos, DVDs, and a detailed guide. DVDs may include extra tracks. For example, the DVD for *Love's Passion* has an alternate soundtrack of commentary by Veronica Hart and the female lead, Juli Ashton. The casual girlfriends-discussing-porn dialogue may be more of a turn-on than the original soundtrack.

You can also call Good Vibrations at 1-800-289-8423 for a catalogue (know that you will keep getting their catalogues in the mail). The catalogues are discreetly packaged, but not something you want to open with your kids watching.

Since videos cost $30 to $50, you'll want a good sense of what you're buying before you commit. I know that seems like a lot of money for an experiment, but keep in mind that if this works, you'll think it's a bargain compared to a bottle of wine. Good Vibrations (Web and print catalogue) classifies its merchandise according to eleven categories, including woman-centered, strong plot, multicultural, and whether the film has a heterosexual, gay, or lesbian theme.

Play Wisely

A critical privacy need for parents is a separate space that locks. This might be a tool box, a filing cabinet, a desk drawer, or wicker basket with a lock that fits over the latch, kept in a closet or under the bed. Store the key to the lock on each parent's key chain (don't underestimate your teenager's creativity or curiosity). Without certainty that you can have inaccessible space for storage, you won't be comfortable with exploring some of the options mentioned here.

Games and Playfulness

Sexual games are essentially the opposite of sexual mindfulness. Sexual games are, by definition, intentional, structured or semistructured, and premeditated. Some playfulness can be incorporated into parental quickie sex, while others will require the rare private space and time that you may get only occasionally. Consider these erotic forays in place of lovemaking, something you can do for ten or fifteen minutes one night when you're too tired or sleep deprived for more.

One of the most common sexual games that you might wish to try is to blindfold each other. You can buy a faux fur or leather blindfold for under $20 at any online sex shop (such as www.libida.com). Or use a scarf (or just promise to keep your eyes closed) and explore sensory sensations. Part of what is erotic about this is the heightened tactile awareness that comes from removing the visual sense, and part is simply that it is erotic to be intentional, unconventional, vulnerable, and/or in control. You can simply let the moment guide you and explore his body with your own.

You can add structure by asking him to guess what you're using to touch him (try a cotton ball, a feather, a warm washcloth, light strokes with a hairbrush, or whatever is at hand). Spell words on his skin using your finger or a Q-tip. If you're short on time, remember that you can do this without moving on to intercourse. It's a perfect way to spread lovemaking out over a few days by trading turns.

Another game is to pretend that you are teenagers trying to hide sex from your parents. The only cost here is the baby-sitter. Whatever you did before when the last place on earth that you could fool around at was your house, do again. It might mean spending some time in the backseat of the car or checking into a motel for a few hours like you did in college. Instead of being annoyed by the lack of opportunity, get back in touch with the aphrodisiac of sneaking around.

The next shopping trip is to a place you know well: the grocery store. Making love with food is another very common fantasy. This one almost certainly requires the kids to be at Grandma's, but the grocery checkout clerk won't bat an eye when you leave the store with a bottle of champagne and some chocolate sauce. Try popcorn: Take a popcorn kernel, place one in an interesting place, and nibble it. If you get caught with popcorn in your bedroom, your kids won't think twice, but be sure to put the chocolate sauce or whipped cream back in the refrigerator.

Combine taste with touch. Bring a Popsicle to the bedroom and warm up spots you've just made cold. I'd advise against using food inside your vagina, since this can increase the risk of a bladder infection. Urinate immediately after if you do play with food internally or near either partner's urethral opening (the tube to the bladder).

Another sexual game that couples may enjoy taps into fantasies about voyeurism, exhibitionism, and vulnerability: taking photographs while making love. While you're at the grocery store or pharmacy, pick up a disposable Polaroid camera ($20). Agree in advance that the photographs will be destroyed (or kept only if you have a childproof storage system that rivals Fort Knox and you *both* want to keep them). The eroticism is in the process, and a pair of scissors and good plumbing is all it takes to get rid of the evidence. Do not allow even the possibility that your kids could find the photographs. You don't want to have that conversation.

If you are interested but feel too shy to bring up one of these ideas to your husband, try easing into it. One way to check out his reaction is to present the idea as something you stumbled over. For example, if he knows you're reading this book, show him this page, and open the discussion with a neutral comment: "What do you think of what Dr. Raskin suggests here?"

Another way to ease into the discussion of sexual playfulness is to order the catalogue Red Envelope (on line at www.redenvelope.com or 1-877-333-6836). This catalogue is primarily a very conventional Lillian Vernon–ish catalogue of corporate gifts, children's items, jewelry, and gardening gadgets, but it also happens to include a few romantic adventure items nestled in (including body dice as described below). It's perfect for saying "Look at what I found next to the gourmet gingersnaps." If he recoils in horror, move on. If he seems at all intrigued, open the dialogue.

You can also find not-too-kinky games in catalogues and on the Web (see the listings for vibrators). Several sites sell versions of dice that you could make yourself with Scotch tape, a set of dice, and paper and pencil. Include one die that lists body parts (be as oblique as you wish; "above the waist" is good enough), an erotic verb ("caress," "taste," "warm"). Roll and play. Other common games available include edible finger paint and flavored body powders (such as "honey dust").

Let your imagination guide you. Just as fantasies are uniquely your own, you may have all sorts of ideas for how to make your love-making more varied. Or he may, but perhaps has been waiting for permission. For more ideas, pick up Joan Elizabeth Lloyd's *52 Saturday Nights: Heat Up Your Sex Life Even More with a Year of Creative Lovemaking* (Warner, 2000).

Vibrators

If you haven't tried a vibrator, consider it. Three main issues keep women from considering purchasing a vibrator. The first is the feeling that it isn't natural or "shouldn't be necessary." It isn't natural or necessary, but neither is a candlelight dinner, high-heeled shoes, or fancy lingerie. A vibrator is simply an alternative that can greatly increase the likelihood of either having an orgasm or having a really intense one. When sex is more physically pleasurable, you want more of it. It's an excellent option for increasing libido by increasing the "reward." Wouldn't we expect that men would be less interested in sex if climax were less predictable or as much of an effort as it often is for women?

A vibrator is the most widely recommended medical treatment for women who aren't having orgasms, because it works.[1]

---

[1] Interestingly, physicians used vibrators for medical treatment of "female hysteria" as early as the 1800s. Prior to that, midwives recommended orgasm, which they believed enhanced fertility. See Rachel P. Maines, *The Technology of Orgasm: Hysteria, the Vibrator and Women's Sexual Satisfaction* (Baltimore: Johns Hopkins University Press, 2001), for a fascinating history of the vibrator.

The second concern many women have, especially those who have tried a vibrator during times without an available sexual partner, is that it can become "addictive." The concern is that it is so easy to climax with a vibrator that you won't be able to climax without one. Although most women's sexual literature dismisses this concern, I believe there is some foundation to it. You won't become addicted in the true sense of the word. A vibrator won't make you forsake carpooling or your job while you pleasure yourself in the bedroom. However, some women do notice that a very intense orgasm, such as that induced by a vibrator, leaves them temporarily refractory (physically insensitive) to further orgasms unless the physical stimulation is extremely intense, à la another vibrator-induced climax. It won't be an issue for women who have several days or a week between lovemaking, and it won't ever be an issue if you use it only intermittently.

If you do find that a highly predictable, intense orgasm is an option you always choose, that's not addiction, that's making a sexual choice. Some perfectly sexually normal women use vibrators every time they make love and find that it enhances their sexual relationship by taking the pressure of will-she-or-won't-she-climax off both partners.[2] Some women are able to use vibrators freely interspersed with equipment-free orgasms, although these may be women who are very easily orgasmic in the first place. In all cases, if you find that you don't like how using a vibrator affects subsequent sexual experiences, which may feel like "addiction," simply stop using it and your body will definitely return to pre-vibrator sensitivity within a short time. Sexual refractoriness is never "permanent."

The third issue is the discomfort of acquiring and owning a vibra-

[2]A vibrator is one of my first suggestions for patients taking sex-killing antidepressants, since the serotonin increase caused by these medications greatly lowers sexual sensitivity and responsiveness. It's also a great idea for women who are avoiding hormone replacement therapy for menopause, or who haven't found that hormones restore physical sexual responsiveness.

tor. All mothers should have a locked private place to store anything they want to keep away from the children. Getting a vibrator can be a private matter. Drugstores, discount chains, and health stores typically sell body massagers designed for nonsexual use: relaxation, muscle aches, or sports injury rehabilitation. These can be used for sexual purposes. Of course, if you check out with KY Jelly, condoms, and a vibrator, expect a raised eyebrow. If you throw some diapers and Disney Band-Aids in the cart, you can count on the cashier's moms-don't-have-sex stereotypic thinking to make the transaction quite comfortable.

Better yet, the Web has made access to vibrators remarkably easy and private. You can get vibrators at online drugstores as well as women-operated sex sites. The shipping boxes are discreet, although if your children are like mine, they'll ask about what's in the box, hoping it's for them. Have a bland response ready. Cost runs from under $10 to over $100, with an average price between $20 to $30. They truly come in all shapes, sizes, colors, and textures. Each of the following three online stores also offers an 800 number for ordering. They are:

Toys in Babeland, www.babeland.com, 1-800-658-9119

Good Vibrations, www.goodvibes.com, 1-800-289-8423

Eve's Garden, www.evesgarden.com, 1-800-848-3837.

Candida Royalle also sells her own line of vibrators, Natural Contours, at www.royalle.com.html, 1-800-456-5683. You can also find "personal massagers" that you could give to your grandmother for her arthritis at www.drugstore.com, Kmart's online store, www.bluelight.com, or go upscale at www.sharperimage.com.

How to choose? First, let me warn you that all of the erotic store sites listed above, while woman-operated, may be offensive to some. They are explicit, include photographs and drawings of the merchandise, and all sell items targeted at a very wide audience (you can get cuffs, neon dildos, and nipple clips, too). Others will find the sites as exciting as the best erotic video or story and may like perusing the online catalogues for fun. You'll notice that most vibrators look like bizarre phallic symbols. Some are very realistically shaped to resemble a penis, many in colors and sizes not found in nature.

If you like a big neon-blue battery-operated phallus, you can find it. I'm going to steer you toward the alternatives that won't scream "kinky sex." All three sites offer staff advice about the products, and the Babes in Toyland site has a "vibe coach" that takes you through a decision tree to sort through the options.

The basic decision besides cost is electric vs. battery operated. Electric vibrators are more powerful, often quieter, but less geographically flexible than the battery-operated models. However, electric vibrators are usually also sold for medical purposes such as shoulder pain, and so may be more appealing to the discreet buyer. Don't use the heat setting on these medical models, and don't go near water with an electric vibrator.[3]

A very popular new line of battery vibrators has been developed by Candida Royalle, available at several of the Web sites mentioned above, as well as www.drugstore.com, called Natural Contours. All of these sites show photographs, and you'll see that they are a nice, discreet alternative to a hard metal tropical-colored phallic vibrator. The makers claim that even the airport security detectors won't realize what that thing in your purse is for.

Two vibrators that may be more appealing to couples are designed for human touch. The first and oldest model is the Wahl Swedish-style massager, which is an electric vibrator that goes over the hand

---

[3]There are specific battery-operated vibrators available at these sites designed for use in water. One brand name is the Aquassager, or look for the term "waterproof."

like a bionic glove. It transmits vibration through your partner's fingers. The newest and very popular variation is the Fukuoku 9000, which is a small watch-battery operated vibrator that goes over the fingertip (and I'm not making up the name!). These are less intensely stimulating but often feel more erotically stimulating or integrated because they simply augment natural touch.

It's Supposed to Be Fun

All of these ideas are merely suggestions. People make love in many different ways, and it's worth considering what others have found to be enjoyable. An occasional foray into new territory will help you overcome the sexual blahs, but it doesn't make any sense to try anything that interferes with being relaxed during lovemaking. Stay in your comfort zone or, better yet, inch ever so slightly outside of it. Keep a sense of humor, and remember that sex is supposed to be fun.

Affirmation
"When choosing between two evils, I always like to try the one I've never tried before."
—Mae West

Step Ten: Take Help from the Experts

"... there are few cures in medicine, with the exception of antibiotics, but there is help and improvement."

—Judith Reichman, M.D., *I'm Not in the Mood: What Every Woman Should Know About Improving Her Libido*

- Substituting alternative medications may help women experiencing sexual side effects of common prescriptions, including antidepressants and blood pressure medicines.
- Appropriate treatment of endocrine and other physiological conditions that can impact sexuality can have a dramatically beneficial effect.
- Talk therapy alternatives include sex therapy, couples therapy, and individual therapy.

If you've worked your way through the first nine steps, and things still aren't right sexually, it's time to figure out whether something is in need of professional repair. On the other hand, if you're starting with this chapter, you've missed my sermons about how there usually isn't a quick fix for unsatisfying sex in parents raising kids. It takes a good deal of time and effort to overcome a lifetime's cultural misinformation, years of hurt or miscommunication, sexual shyness, and longstanding bad habits.

Depending on your perspective, that's either good or bad news. It's bad news if you're hoping for a pill or a cream that would make everything the way it used to be, even if your doctor has shrugged and told you, "Sorry, nothing I can do." It's good news if you've already had every blood test in the universe, and you're relieved that you won't have to take medicine. It's also good news if you know that sexual difficulties can be blessings in disguise, opportunities to make things even better than they were before.

I learned this early in my career as a psychiatrist. I was treating a woman with postpartum obsessive-compulsive disorder (OCD). The only effective medications for OCD increase serotonin in the body as well as the brain, which, unfortunately, lowers sex drive and makes climax very difficult if not impossible. My patient, a mother of two small children, had a fantastic response to Prozac for her OCD symptoms. Unfortunately, the same medication that helped her feel like herself emotionally destroyed her sexual response, and she asked for my help. She was in a catch-22: If we lowered the dose or changed medicine, her sexual side effects improved, but the OCD flared up. I tried a series of medicines designed to overcome this side effect, with little impact.

Just when I was ready to throw in the towel, she breezed into my office and joyfully announced that her problem was solved: Her husband changed his sexual technique. Instead of rushing to the end zone, they created the time for leisurely lovemaking, and she went from being bored to fully engaged in lovemaking. She told me that Prozac was the best thing that ever happened to her. As a couple, they made lemonade out of lemons. Until things completely shut down sexually, they hadn't really paid attention to how things had gradually declined since the kids were born, truthfully, well before the Prozac was even an issue.

As useful a lesson as this was for me, I want to be sure that we're not too quick to dismiss medical causes or medical treatment as an option. Women's sexuality is terribly neglected in the pharmaceutical and medical profession, and physicians are way too quick to conclude that loss of sex drive or sexual pleasure is an inevitable result of aging, femaleness, or managing an illness. Other physicians never got enough training to become comfortable talking about sexual concerns, even if they know what to do about the problem. Three of the ten most commonly prescribed medications in America (Prozac, Paxil, and Zoloft) wreak havoc on sexuality, and mainstream medicine has been extremely slow to tune into the importance of reversible causes of sexual dysfunction in women.

In this chapter, we'll consider four possible ways to professionally repair what's still not working right. These include: 1) the possibility that you're taking a medication that is harming your sex life; 2) possible physiological conditions that can cause sexual dysfunction and explore medical options that might help; 3) the first FDA-approved sexual medical device for women; and 4) types of talk therapy that can repair sexual, emotional, and relational problems.

Medications with Sexual Side Effects

Sexual side effects of medications might include lowered sex drive, changes in orgasm, or decreased lubrication, which can cause discomfort during lovemaking. The hallmark of a medication-induced sexual side effect is any noticeable change in sexual function or pleasure that begins within the first few weeks of starting or raising the dose of the prescription. It's easy to tell when you've been warned in advance by your physician that sexual side effects are possible, but much harder to tell when you haven't been warned to look for it. Trust your instincts, and don't let your physician dismiss your concerns or questions.

If you find that your physician doesn't take your concerns seriously, you must take charge of your own body. Doctors generally concern themselves first and foremost with successful treatment of a condition: Does the medicine do what it's supposed to do (e.g., lower blood pressure, ameliorate depression)? Your goal as a patient is to find a treatment that is better than the illness, a medication with acceptable side effects.

No medication is side-effect free, so sexual dysfunction is sometimes an unavoidable situation, but you should *never* assume that you have no reasonable medical alternatives to giving up your sex life. If sexual side effects are unavoidable, you must ask your doctor to help you find ways to overcome the side effects, which might include comedication, or using a second medication to "treat" the side effects.

Be as active a consumer with your physician as you would be if the patient were your child. Insist on enough time to discuss the topic. Talk to the office nurse before your appointment to alert the doctor (which may give him or her a chance to review scientific information on the side effect). Do your own Web search and come in with information that supports your self-diagnosis. Don't succumb to the fear of authority, to the doctor's nonverbal messages of being too busy, or to anyone's discomfort talking about sexuality. You may need to find a new doctor if yours isn't concerned with helping you manage this side effect.

If you have started a medication and noticed a change in sexual function, assume that there is a connection unless proven otherwise. If you aren't sure, ask your doctor and expect a thoughtful answer. Bear in mind that if these medications are prescribed for your husband, he may have similar problems with arousal and sex drive, and may also have erectile dysfunction or changes in orgasm, including inability to climax.

If you find that something you are taking is on the list of medicines known to cause sexual side effects, do not taper or stop the medication without medical supervision. The consequences of stopping medication without your doctor's guidance and approval could be dangerous or life-threatening.

The following medications are particularly prone to causing sexual side effects:

Antidepressants (which may be prescribed for depression, panic disorder, anxiety disorders, social phobia, obsessive-compulsive disorder and premenstrual dysphoric disorder). The worst culprits are those medications that increase serotonin, which is a sexually inhibitory chemical in the brain as well as the body. These include Prozac, Zoloft, Paxil, Celexa, Effexor, Luvox, and Anafranil. Most other psychiatric medications can cause sexual side effects, although the above are the most likely by far. For more information, I refer you to my book *When Words Are Not Enough: The Women's Prescription for Depression and Anxiety* (Broadway Books, 1997).

Antihypertensives (which may be prescribed for lowering blood pressure; heart disease including heart rhythm disturbances, congestive heart failure, or hardening of the arteries; migraine headaches; and fluid retention, including PMS). These medications, including diuretics (hydrochlorthiazide), beta blockers (Corgard, Lopressor, Tenormin), and the old-fashioned medications such as reserpine and methyldopa, may reduce libido and cause sexual dysfunction. Calcium channel blockers (Cardizem, Procardia, Norvasc) or ACE inhibitors (Vasotec, Zestril) may be a better alternative.

Anxiolytics (most commonly prescribed for anxiety disorders and insomnia). These include Xanax (alprazolam), Ativan (lorazepam), Klonopin (clonazepam), and numerous others. They usually do not cause inability to climax, but may reduce libido. BuSpar is an alternative for some anxiety disorders, and Ambien and Sonata are alternative sleeping medications.

Birth control pills. There is little clear information on the impact of birth control pills on libido, even though they clearly reduce sex drive in many women. Birth control pills generally do not have any negative effect on climax. However, since the estrogen component of oral contraceptives stimulates production of the protein that binds testosterone, it makes less available freely circulating testosterone, a major hormonal component of libido in both sexes. Making matters worse, the newest forms of synthetic progesterone in birth control pills may bring about an additional libido plunge, because they lack the testosterone-mimicking quality that natural and older synthetic progestins have (called their androgenic component). On the other hand, sometimes the estrogen sexual tradeoff is that you often have better vaginal lubrication, which may make sex more enjoyable.

These counteracting sexual side effects may mean that the only way to figure out what is best for you is by trial and error, substituting one type of pill for what you're currently taking and comparing the different side effects. Some women find that taking an oral contraceptive that contains the older progestin called norethindrone at a dose of 1.5 nanograms helps restore the proper balance for libido. Another alternative is the so-called mini-pill, which contains no estrogen.

Hormone replacement therapy (HRT) (estrogen, estrogen plus progestin, and estrogen patches). Hormone replacement has generally been an option at surgical or natural menopause, to reduce the risk of osteoporosis, heart disease, hot flashes, etc. The estrogen component of HRT helps reduce vaginal dryness and atrophy, which makes sexual intercourse more enjoyable. But some women notice that HRT's beneficial effect on libido soon wears off. That is because estrogen triggers production of a protein that binds testosterone, effectively lowering your natural libido-boosting hormone.

An alternative that may be appropriate for some women is a form of HRT that includes testosterone, such as Estratest or Estratest H.S. Women who are taking HRT after surgical menopause (for example, if your ovaries were removed during a hysterectomy), are especially good candidates for including testosterone with HRT. More about the pros and cons of testosterone later.

Over-the-counter medications can cause sexual side effects, too. Cold, allergy, and analgesic medications with the term "PM" (e.g., Tylenol-PM), and nonprescription sleeping medications typically contain antihistamines that can cause vaginal dryness and thereby make sex uncomfortable. Over-the-counter antacids (also available in prescription strength) such as Pepcid and Tagamet can reduce libido.

Is It the Underlying Disease?

Although medications used for the conditions described above can have sexual side effects, it is often difficult to determine whether the condition being treated is part of the problem. Libido-killing medication is most frequently prescribed for depression and high blood pressure, but if untreated, these conditions can squelch libido on their own; for example, high blood pressure may reduce pelvic blood flow.

Depression itself is associated with low sex drive, and it may be hard to sort out how much of the problem is due to the illness rather than the treatment. The key question is whether the low libido came along with the symptoms of depression (see next box) or followed medical treatment for depression with an antidepressant. You have the absolute right to advice and support from your personal physician in exploring the underlying cause of your sexual difficulty and in seeking treatment options that preserve your sexual pleasure.

Clinical depression is the illness most likely to cause low libido in mothers. When five or more of the following symptoms are present most or all of the day for two weeks or longer, the individual may be experiencing clinical depression:

- sad or empty mood,
- loss of enjoyment in things one used to find pleasurable,
- hopelessness,
- insomnia or excessive sleeping,
- appetite or weight changes,
- anxiety or panic attacks,
- poor concentration,
- low self-esteem,
- guilty feelings,
- thoughts of suicide or escape,
- low energy.

Many other illnesses contribute to low sex drive or lowered responsiveness. In general, fatigue itself, a common aspect of a wide variety of conditions, can make you too tired for sex. More specifically, diseases that might reduce blood flow or nerve supply to the pelvis (diabetes, cardiovascular disease, pelvic surgery or radiation, lung disease), hormone imbalances (especially thyroid, adrenal, ovarian hormone deficiencies, including testosterone), autoimmune diseases, cancer, and chronic pain can affect sensation, engorgement, lubrication, or orgasm. Smoking and alcohol abuse can also cause sexual dysfunction.

Gynecologist Judith Reichman's book *(I'm Not in the Mood)* and urologist Jennifer Berman's coauthored book, *For Women Only: A*

Revolutionary Guide to Overcoming Sexual Dysfunction and Reclaiming Your Life are outstanding medical references, which may include more information about medical causes and treatments for female sexual dysfunction than your doctor knows. The next box lists medical tests that diagnose common physiological causes of low libido.

Routine blood tests for medical causes of low libido should include:

- CBC (complete blood count) to rule out anemia
- TSH to rule out hypothyroidism
- Free testosterone level

Depending on age and other clinical symptoms, other blood tests might include:

- Prolactin level to rule out pituitary disease
- DHEA-S to measure adrenal function
- FSH to diagnose menopause

Usually, people find it reassuring to know that they don't have a serious medical problem. We'd all rather have "stress" cause our headaches than a brain tumor. When it comes to sex, however, that's often not the case. Many women would like to have something to pin it on and, surprisingly, some are disappointed when a testosterone test, for example, comes back normal. Try to keep self-judgment out of the diagnostic arena. If you have low libido with otherwise picture-perfect health, you aren't any less genuinely afflicted than a person with a diagnosed medical cause. Likewise, having a diagnosable condition or taking a medication that causes sexual side effects doesn't mean that you don't have a responsibility to be as sexually assertive, intentional, brave, and creative as anyone else! Even clearly medically based sexual symptoms may respond to changes in how you make love.

Is There Something I Can Take?

One reason to have a medical workup for low libido is to find out whether there is a specific treatment to correct the problem. If there is a clear medical cause, medicine, if tolerated (any time you take something, you risk a new set of side effects), will usually help. Other treatments may help even in the absence of a known chemical problem, just as Viagra (sildenafil) helps some men with erectile function whether or not they have a problem of aging or a diagnosed medical problem such as diabetes.

It isn't possible to say with scientific certainty that there is any medication, herb, or vitamin that enhances sexual responsiveness or function in women that is equivalent to Viagra for men. A pill that you think will improve your sex life may improve your sex life just because you think it will, a phenomenon called the placebo effect. The placebo effect is what makes generalizing from another person's story about how a particular cream or pill caused a mind-blowing orgasm anything but scientific. Making matters more complicated, many studies that investigate treatment of sexual difficulties in women throw everything under the sun into the study.

This issue is especially pertinent to trying to figure out what role if any Viagra has in women. Viagra promotes genital vascular congestion in men and women alike, hence its role in erectile dysfunction ("impotence") in men. The value for women isn't established. The studies have been disappointing, suggesting that Viagra is no more effective than placebo for women. However, unlike the more homogeneous population of men studied, the studies for women have thrown women with histories of childhood sexual abuse together with women who were fine until they started taking an antidepressant. I believe it is quite possible that when studies are conducted with a carefully selected group of women (those with a clear chemical or vascular component contributing to anorgasmia), Viagra will be shown to be effective. In my own practice, with the patient's informed consent, I've successfully prescribed Viagra for women suffering anorgasmia due to psychiatric medication. Drs. Berman describe similar clinical success in their book.

Other medications available by prescription are at early stages of investigation or clinical use, and I discourage you from being too quick to jump on the bandwagon. This is especially so because, as has been true for Viagra, the studies will be conducted on men first. What works for men won't automatically translate to women, and potential side effects won't be the same. If you are considering taking a medication to promote sexual responsiveness, I urge you to seek out a specialist. That said, there is growing evidence that the following available or forthcoming medications may promote return or ease of climax: phentolamine, apomorphine, prostaglandin E-1 cream, and bupropion (Wellbutrin or Zyban).

Unless there is a strong link between inability to climax and low sex drive, the above medications won't usually promote sexual interest. Hormones are more effective for low libido, but it isn't clear whether they have any benefit in the absence of a diagnosed deficiency. However, as noted by Susan Rako, M.D., psychiatrist and author of *The Hormone of Desire: The Truth About Testosterone, Sexuality and Menopause* (Three Rivers Press, 1999), medical laboratory references only list *excessive* testosterone as abnormal, neglecting to identify the population of testosterone-deficient women. Because the ovaries slow their production of testosterone at menopause, testosterone deficiency is interpreted as "normal," i.e., not excessive.

Ask your doctor to show you the test results and explain whether your "normal" was *within* the normal range, *or simply less than* the laboratory-defined upper limit. There is a growing consensus that there is such a thing as too little testosterone and that replacing testosterone in diagnosed deficiency, or adding it to HRT, often reverses low libido. Lowish levels of testosterone (at the lowest end of the spectrum of the lab's value for normal) may respond to treatment as well and certainly warrant a repeat test six months later. Along with low libido, symptoms of testosterone deficiency can include fatigue, headaches, dryness in hair and skin, and muscle atrophy.

When a woman's testosterone level is low, the impact of normalizing it is very dramatic. Most women with low libido have normal testosterone; most of the time, when I test for testosterone in my patients, the results are perfectly normal. Unfortunately, some women can't take testosterone due to other medical problems (such as liver disease); others don't want to risk or put up with the masculinizing side effects (such as acne and facial hair). The potential risk of cardiovascular disease due to raised cholesterol and serum lipids (fats) caused by these tiny doses of testosterone remains medically controversial. Your doctor can compare a pre- and post-testosterone fasting lipid profile to monitor for this possible adverse effect of testosterone.

Other endocrine deficiencies that cause treatable low libido include DHEA (dehydroepiandrosterone) and thyroid deficiency. The benefit of DHEA, available over the counter, for women with normal DHEA levels is unclear and controversial. Although available without prescription, DHEA is not without side effects, including masculinization.

A generally safe and very promising natural alternative is gingko biloba, which has been used in herbal medicine for centuries. Recent medical studies have shown that gingko increases small blood vessel flow, which has given it a minor role in helping to slow the progression of Alzheimer's dementia. Gingko has also been shown to help men with erectile dysfunction and both women and men who have experienced sexual side effects of antidepressants, presumably by the same mechanism. My warning about anecdotal evidence notwithstanding, I've had a good deal of success in my patients. One recent study indicated that a combination of gingko with ginseng promoted sexual desire in women. These herbs are generally well tolerated and worth giving a month or two trial to see if libido or threshold of climax improves. It doesn't seem to work unless taken regularly, and some women find that the doses needed (100 to 200 mg or more) can cause unacceptable gastrointestinal distress. The only serious but very rare side effect of ginkgo is easy bruising, and it is unsafe for women taking blood thinners such as warfarin (Coumadin), or regular aspirin.

A Medical Device for Female Sexual Pleasure

The FDA recently approved a new medical approach to inability to climax or inadequate sexual arousal. It's a device called the Eros Therapy (originally named the Eros-CTD). The good news: Eros Therapy helps many, not all, women with female sexual dysfunction (FSD) experience more clitoral sensation, better lubrication, and achieve orgasm more readily. Studies indicate that women with FSD who use the device also report increased sexual satisfaction overall.

Eros Therapy is a battery-operated handheld device about the size of a transistor radio with a small plastic cup that goes over the clitoris. When you turn it on, the device provides gentle suction to the clitoris. This stimulates blood flow and clitoral engorgement, which increases lubrication and sensation. It may sound alarming to imagine your clitoris being suctioned, but if you've ever used a breast pump for milk, you know that gentle suction to a delicate part of the body is not dangerous or painful. The degree of suction is much gentler, and not only doesn't feel bad, it feels good. It's the *only* mechanical alternative to a vibrator, and differs in that it provides suction (mimicking oral sex) rather than application of stimulation by a vibrator. Like a vibrator, it's safe.

Although Eros Therapy may be especially useful for women with a medical or physiological cause of diminished pleasure (such as diabetes, medication side effects, postsurgical sexual dysfunction, or postmenopausal difficulties) it also is a great alternative for women who have not climaxed previously. Not surprisingly, some studies indicate that women with no sexual problems whatsoever also report increased sensation, ease of climax, and sexual satisfaction.

The bad news: It costs about $300 per device, and it's available only by medical prescription. Your insurance will often cover the cost if your doctor prescribes it and uses the diagnosis of FSD to justify the prescription. If you can afford the device without using your insurance, you'll still need a prescription, but you may have fewer anonymous insurance coders and billers in your private business. If you decide to return the Eros Therapy within 60 days, the company currently offers a full refund.

Some physicians are unfamiliar with Eros Therapy. You can call the company for information at 1-877-774-1442, or download information from www.urometrics.com/products/eros/ and bring it to your doctor when you make the request. Some women are more comfortable discussing the issue with a nurse before the appointment, so that when the doctor comes into the examining room, he or she already knows what issue you'd like to discuss.

Using Eros Therapy is just like using a vibrator: You can do it alone or with a partner. The device comes with a very clear and comprehensive set of instructions, and I recommend that my patients get comfortable using it alone before including it in lovemaking. Once you know how to operate the device (it's quite simple), you can show him. If you want to explore it with a partner, and I encourage you to find the gumption, there is no way to do so without face-to-face discussion. Women who have had a loss of sexual functioning and many who just never fully enjoyed lovemaking often find that their partners are delighted to use the device. Your sexual pleasure matters to your partner, and it's great for both of you.

The Role of Talk Therapy

I urge you to consider some form of talk therapy if you are considering taking medication to enhance your sex drive or pleasure, just as I would argue that a combination of talk therapy and medication is the best treatment for serious clinical depression. Talk therapy may be helpful under the following circumstances: 1) you've tried the self-help suggestions in this book and things are still bad; 2) you or your husband has a specific sexual disorder (it isn't just the blahs); 3) you realize that the problem isn't sexual, it's marital; 4) a history of sexual trauma is contributing to your difficulties (anyone with childhood sexual abuse and many adult rape victims may experience lingering problems of sexual intimacy); 5) you're considering divorce or separation; 6) depression is part of the problem; or 7) you just want to try it (therapy doesn't require justification, except to the HMO, and that is your therapist's job).

Choices for therapy include individual therapy, couples counseling (also called marital therapy), and sex therapy (typically, both members of the couple attend). Individual therapy may be the best place to start if you have a form of depression or posttraumatic stress disorder, because these conditions can cause sexual problems in a couple that is otherwise doing well. Couples counseling is designed to improve relationship communication and build emotional intimacy. Sex therapy often involves more specific sex education and behavioral approaches to sexual dysfunction. In practice, the two are often blended. Although traditional sex therapy is usually reserved for couples, many sex therapists will treat individuals, especially if there is a history of sexual trauma.

The Role of Individual Therapy in Repair

Talk therapy is an effective treatment for the most common cause of low libido: depression. Mood disorders are twice as common in women as men, and the postpartum period is an extremely vulnerable time. Low libido is a common symptom of depression in women, and depression robs you of the energy, hopefulness, and sense of personal efficacy that you need to overcome sexual difficulties. Postpartum depression is not a natural consequence of childbirth, and you shouldn't put off treatment thinking that it will go away on its own. Non-postpartum depression can strike at any vulnerable time. Other reproductive vulnerable times include pregnancy and perimenopause. Nonreproductive transitions include loss, social isolation, caretaker and parenting stress, and divorce. However, you don't need an identifiable cause of depression to respond to talk therapy, or medication therapy, for depression.

Post-traumatic stress disorder (PTSD) may be caused by sexual abuse in childhood or sexual assault (including attempted rape). One of the cardinal symptoms of PTSD is that the victim attempts to avoid memories of the trauma, which is obviously a very significant problem in lovemaking, even when you love your sexual partner. If you have active sexual problems that could be related to past trauma, seek professional help. Your life can change.

Individual therapy can be helpful for a wide variety of emotional factors that can contribute to maternal sexual unhappiness. If you've tried to make your own needs a priority and just can't seem to do it on your own, therapy may help. If you can't conquer the demon of perfectionism, therapy may help. If you grew up with terrible messages about female sexuality, therapy may help. If your husband refuses to go to counseling or sex therapy, individual therapy may help you solve what you can on your own, and it can even help you be more effective in enlisting his involvement in treatment down the road.

How Couples Counseling Can Repair Sexual Problems

Marital therapy works for many sexual problems. Many apparent sexual problems are actually relationship issues, as described in the obstacle "Disconnection" (see page 46). Also, many couples (or one of the spouses) find the idea of marital therapy less intimidating than "sex therapy." Marital therapy is useful for relationship building, improving communication, learning to tolerate differences and changes within each partner, dealing with anger and power issues, conflicts about child rearing, and deepening emotional intimacy. Generally, couples see a therapist once weekly for a period of months or even years.

Couples therapy is often very useful for couples in which one or both members lack a model of successful marriage, either because their parents divorced during their childhood or because their parents remained married but modeled everything that doesn't work in marriage.

Short of formal counseling, consider a weekend retreat for marriage building. Many churches, synagogues, and family life centers offer marriage workshops (sometimes called marriage encounter weekends, marriage enrichment, or marriage seminars) designed to strengthen marriages that aren't necessarily or obviously at risk. You take your car in for maintenance, and it doesn't mean the car is defective. Why not a marriage tuneup? To locate one, search the Web or ask your clergyperson. (Be aware that some marriage workshops have a politically conservative mission to make wives more submissive, but most do not.)

Sex Therapy

Sex therapy may be useful for sexual boredom, although it is usually reserved for specific types of sexual dysfunction. If you or your husband has a specific sexual problem that hasn't been addressed by this book, you may wish to seek treatment from a sex therapist. Appendix B describes the classification system used by the American Psychiatric Association to describe subtypes of sexual dysfunction.

Standard sex therapy doesn't ignore relationship issues, but certified sex therapists generally have specialized training and skills in using behavioral and cognitive interventions for sexual disorders in addition to traditional talk therapy. Sex therapists are generally "ordinary" therapists (social workers, psychologists, marriage counselors, or psychiatrists), who are also expert in sexual physiology, development, and particular techniques. Good sex therapists do not overemphasize the mechanics of sex, and sex therapy never involves anything but talk during the sex therapy session (you won't be asked to undress, bring in photographs, or demonstrate anything sexual in the session).

Most sex therapists will begin by taking a history of the problem that brings you to treatment, how the sexual issue is affecting each member at present, and will probably have you complete a written or verbal sexual developmental history. Typically, sex therapists will assess for potential contributing physiological problems and look at how your upbringing affected each of you. A common first step "prescribed" in sex therapy is a series of exercises and homework called "sensate focus." The therapist often instructs the couple to stop having intercourse initially, to immediately remove the pressure and de-escalate conflict. This is combined with progressively erotic exercises that enhance sexual communication and physical pleasure while deemphasizing intercourse.

Sex therapists typically assign homework exercises that promote sensual reconnection in the privacy of your bedroom. Many parents simply cannot find the time (the usual prescription for homework is for a half hour four or five times per week of sensual touching and massage without intercourse). I've modified this approach for time-starved parents in Step Six, but you should know that the more you practice at home, the better it will work for you. If your therapist refuses to believe that time is an issue, he or she may not be parent-sensitive enough to be helpful. However, don't use time shortage as an excuse for resisting treatment. Try to negotiate a parent-sensitive approach with your sex therapist, and give it your best effort.

Certification by the American Association of Sex Educators, Counselors and Therapists indicates that a therapist has undergone his or her approved training and examination course. Many capable sex therapists are not certified by this organization but are certified by their professional organization (such as a medical specialty board or other mental health professional guild). A good sex therapist should have a working relationship with a medical professional with expertise in sexual health and medicine, since proper diagnosis is the first step toward proper treatment. A physical examination and some basic laboratory work is a good idea before starting sex therapy.

To read more about what sex therapy is like, I encourage you to read Dr. Domeena Renshaw's book, *Seven Weeks to Better Sex* (Dell

Publishing, 1995). She describes how to modify a standard course of sex therapy in a self-help format, in much greater detail. Her program begins with sexual touching without intercourse, builds sexual and nonsexual communication skills, introduces erotic surprise into the relationship, and has several questionnaires that promote information exchange between partners. She also describes Gestalt techniques and "mimicking," which help readers develop new verbal and nonverbal ways of discussing sexuality. By the fifth week, intercourse resumes. You may wish to follow her prescription exactly and decide to consult a therapist if the course she prescribes doesn't work.

How to Find a Therapist

Increasingly, people locate therapists (whether an individual, couples, or sex therapist) according to their health plan coverage. That's an unfortunate reality, and you know best what your financial options are. Ideally, the best way to find a therapist is by recommendation, especially from your personal physician. Your gynecologist, your husband's urologist, or your primary care physician may be able to recommend the type of therapist you'd like to consult.

If you are essentially relying on a list of "providers" according to your insurance coverage, you may be quite happy with the therapist to whom you are referred. However, whether you get a referral from an HMO, your girlfriend, or your doctor, trust your own judgment and common sense about whether the therapist is a good fit. People tend to stay with the first therapist they see, even when their inner radar registers discomfort. Regardless of whether you're seeing a psychiatrist or a marriage counselor, an individual therapist or a certified sex therapist for couples, you are the best judge of whether this is the person for you. Comfort at the personal level is critical to successful outcome. You will get more out of the work when you feel comfortable and optimistic about the therapist. If you feel that the therapist is not getting your problems, is taking sides in couples counseling, is goofy, unempathic, not very smart, or doesn't understand the reality of life with children, seek another referral.

Good therapists are open to your input about problems you see in the therapy. Others blame you for the difficulties, often saying that therapy is supposed to be uncomfortable. Yes, good therapy can be uncomfortable, because a good therapist expects you to stop doing what you've always been doing. But you should never feel shame, fear, or serious discomfort in treatment. You should always feel that the therapist understands your issues and wants to nurture better, happier choices. You shouldn't feel singled out as the one with the problem, any more than your husband should. If one of you feels picked on, the therapy won't be helpful. A common mistake made in couples counseling is quitting therapy because of a poor therapist, and then deciding that therapy itself isn't going to help. Other couples stay too long when one or both members doesn't feel a good fit with a particular therapist. Be a wise consumer when it comes to mental health. Shop around.

You cannot fix some problems yourself. Some problems are solved more quickly or more effectively with help. Getting professional help is not a failure—it's an opportunity. If you're still stuck sexually, please consider giving yourself the support and guidance of expert individualized treatment. You deserve the best sex you can have.

Affirmation

"There are many ways of going forward, but only one way of standing still."
—Franklin D. Roosevelt

Conclusion
Consolidating Change

"Kosher sex is a journey whose destination is a couple
who feel joined not only by the same roof or children, but
especially through the enjoyment and pleasure they constantly
give each other."

—Shmuley Boteach, *Kosher Sex*

Whether one believes that humans are divinely created, wholly
evolved, or evolved under the guidance of a divine hand, we humans
are perfectly designed for a lifetime of sexual pleasure.

Great sex is intimate sex, and intimacy leads to better sex.
Intimate sex is vulnerable, engaged, nurturing, and absorbing. There
is no denying the unique heat of youthful passion, but we do not
have to accept that as the gold standard. Humans are engineered for
great sex in the long haul, because the best sex is committed sex.
Sharing the work and the joy of raising children doesn't have to crush
your sexuality. The commitment of parenthood offers a foundation
for fully opening up to another human being, for sharing body and
soul, for truly making love. When you harness the incredible power
of sexual trust, sex with a familiar partner will be anything but boring.

Great sex is also mature sex, and maturity leads to better sex.
Mature sex is self-accepting, generous, truthful, cozy, and good-
humored. When we finally grow up enough to discover and assert
our erotic potential, we are rewarded with the elegance and content-
ment that flows from a loving partnership. The longer you make love
with the same person, the more years you have together to integrate

confidence with vulnerability, to stumble and get right back up. The longer you make love as a grown-up, the less you believe in fairy-tales. Making love as a grown-up means rejecting myths, claiming your authentic sexual self, and taking charge.

Great sex is unlike anything else, but it is also just like lots of other things. Like mothering or swimming or baking bread or solving quadratic equations, intimate-sex takes intentionality and practice. Procreation is innate, but making love must be learned, nurtured, and honored. To consolidate changes, keep at it. Try, and then try some more. Let small successes lead to taking bigger risks.

Make the time, find the courage, and reach for the stars.

Affirmation

"The future belongs to those who believe in the beauty of their dreams."

—Eleanor Roosevelt

Appendix A: Sexual Advice for Dads

Many fathers experience a noticeable change in their sex lives after children are born. Just as mothers receive toxic messages about sexuality, so too are men subject to cultural myths and unrealistic expectations about sex. Many parents, moms and dads alike, believe some or all of the contradictory messages about sex, including that everyone else has a better sex life, that kids necessarily destroy your sex life, that Real Men innately know how to please a woman in bed, or that sex is all chemical so there's nothing you can do about it anyway.

True, it's challenging to keep passion alive while meeting the demands of family and work life. And, true, many married couples struggle with the sexual blahs. But sexual blahs are not inevitable. While much of this book is directed at your wife, it is important for you to know that sexuality is a couples issue. She can't fix what's wrong alone any more than you can do so by yourself.

If you have the time, it would be useful to read this book in its entirety. If you can't manage that, I suggest that you focus on Steps 4 and 6, improving sexual communication and making sex more mindful. If that's too much, here's the short version of what I believe husbands need to know about their wives' sexuality.

"Sex tips" evoke the idea of advice on secret spots, special techniques, or ways to fancy up lovemaking. Forget it. The best sex tips for husbands looking to put the spark back in lovemaking are extremely simple. Married, committed, lifelong sexuality is enhanced by a great relationship. Here are sex tips that work:

Court Her Like You Used To

You remember the early days of sizzling sex. We tend to look back on those days and give credit to biology (the newness of the sexual relationship) or to the simpler pace of life (when time wasn't a luxury). Both of these are factors, but chances are that you both paid a lot more attention to courting one another. You remembered to tell her she looked beautiful; she wanted to hear every detail of how your day went at work.

Being the center of the universe of the person you love is incredibly sexy. It's affirming to be chosen and appreciated and romanced. Most parents let this slide. Many husbands feel defensive about being asked to be more romantic, perhaps because they feel criticized for being a guy, or perhaps because it seems silly after all these years.

This isn't about being right or wrong. I can almost guarantee you that if you aren't paying attention to the romantic needs of your wife, she isn't very interested in sex. Male interest is sex is far less linked to relationship needs, and it is baffling to many men that this is how women are. This is how women are. Deal with it. Don't waste another second thinking about whether it's right or fair or logical. Throw yourself into it for three months before deciding it isn't working.

You may also feel awkward or inept about something as vague as "be more romantic." I'm going to spare you the usual advice about bringing flowers or telling her she looks pretty (although I'm in favor of both). If you want concrete advice, pick up Michael Webb's *The RoMANtic's Guide: Hundreds of Creative Tips for a Lifetime of Love* (Hyperion, 2000). Call her in the middle of the day, send an e-card, brush her hair, surprise her with an afternoon out with her best friend while you take the kids, buy little gifts (a box of fancy tea, a nice pen, a blank writing book, a bar of aromatic soap, a sexy CD, anything that lets her know that you think about her in a feminine way when you aren't together), get her car washed, notice and tell her things you like about how she's raising the kids, ask about her day at work. If these seem, well, too sappy, try traditional male stuff: open the door for her, help her with carrying heavy bags, clean the ice off her windshield.

Why are women so affected by these gestures? *Esquire* says it better than I could in their list "Things a Man Should Know About Women," available for your chuckling pleasure at www.esquire.com. My two favorite tips: "An unsolicited kiss is to a woman as free play-off tickets are to a man," and "The quirky perfect gift that shows you've been listening is worth twice the value of anything you can find at Tiffany's." It's being noticed, being nurtured in the little ways that mean so much to us. To women, mothering is about noticing the small details of kids' lives, and romance is about having *our* details noticed. It validates our non-mommy selves, which is the part that both of you want to nourish.

Initiate Sex More Effectively

One of the most frequent complaints I hear from women whose libido lags behind their husbands' is that they feel pressured to have sex. Take an honest look at how you ask for and initiate sex. The most common complaint is entitlement: "He points out how long it's been since the last time." Whether you feel entitled to have sex because it's been twenty-four hours or twenty-four days, asking for sex because of how long it's been is likely to backfire. Women often experience any hint of a request for sex on the basis of not having had sex lately as a personal rejection, proof that you'd do it with any willing vagina.

Instead, ask for sex on the basis of desiring her, not desiring sex. Pay attention to the words you use and be clear that you are attracted to *her*.

Banish the Judge

In couples and/or sex therapy, many couples begin looking for the therapist to proclaim which spouse is "right." It is common to resist changing, because doing something differently feels like giving in, admitting that you are wrong. Try to allow for the possibility of change without either of you being designated as the aggrieved party. Change because it suits you to do so. Go first. Be generous. Assume that whatever you've tried to do to fix the sexual blahs hasn't worked because it isn't working for you two as a couple, not because one of you is hard of hearing or not speaking loudly enough.

She's seeking to do things differently by reading this book. Believe that you need to do so also, and that neither party wins in front of the judge. It isn't about being right, it's about being happy.

Banish the Concept of Foreplay

"Foreplay" emphasizes intercourse and orgasm as the goal of sex, the good stuff that goes after the prologue. An all-too-common football model of sex, which starts with a kickoff and ends with a touchdown, is very alien to most women, especially busy mothers. It contributes to the second most common complaint I hear from women: "not enough affection." The distinction between sex (intercourse/orgasm) and affection (everything else) is a common stumbling block for parents seeking more passion. Men often hear "I need more affection" as criticism ("I need more affection, you big oaf") or as an unwelcome substitute ("I need more affection and a lot less sex"). Mothers often feel as if they have been giving of themselves all day. When they get into bed, they want affection and maybe seduction, but not more demands on their bodies.

In fact, what many women are seeking when they ask for more affection is more sensual touching that may or may not lead to intercourse. A loving wife who is aware that she doesn't want as much sex as her husband often withdraws from physical contact for fear that he'll automatically assume she wants or is agreeing to have sex. This results in women avoiding sensual touching if they don't already know that they are receptive to lovemaking. Since women are generally more receptive after a period of sensual touching, you both lose. Encouraging your wife to feel comfortable engaging in sexual touches without risking your annoyance or disappointment if she decides not to proceed to intercourse will, paradoxically, lead to more intercourse.

This is a bona fide sex tip every sex therapist knows: More erotic touching leads to more sex, even though all erotic touching doesn't and shouldn't. This a simple transformation. Rather than keeping score or track of how often you make love, focus on improving the sensual connection and sexual affection. Good sex is affectionate, and affection is sexy. Get out of the sex/not-sex dichotomy. Kiss more. Hug more. Hold hands more. Almost Do It more.

It may help to understand why your wife both asks for more affection but pulls back from fooling around on the couch. She may believe that she's protecting your male ego by stopping things before they get to the point where she might say no if she doesn't already know that she'll say yes. Culture teaches women that an unconsummated erection is a terrible thing and that giving a man the wrong idea makes one a "tease." Make it clear that you enjoy sensual caresses, kissing, erotic touch, and adolescent fooling around as much as she does.

Don't Believe What They Say About Male Sexuality

It's an open question whether culture is more or less detrimental to men's sexual self-esteem than it is to women's, but it's crystal clear that men also receive many destructive messages about sexuality. One of these is that men should automatically know how to please a woman in bed. As a relationship matures, and the early knock-your-socks-off chemistry wanes, issues of sexual technique may coincide with childbearing and child rearing. What looks like the kids destroying libido is actually an opportunity.

Here's another genuine sex secret: It's okay not to know everything already. Women's bodies are as different as our minds are, and you were not born with telepathy. Take a look at Step 7 for some advice on female erotic geography. Experiment and ask. Try touching new places in new ways, and insist on feedback. Don't believe that a Real Man already knows. Don't believe it is all or even mostly about your penis. Do believe that you have the creativity, imagination, patience, perception, and receptivity to figure out what brings great physical pleasure to your wife. The most important erotic ingredients are neither in a book nor below the waist: your mind, your lips and hands, and your ability to ask and listen.

Likewise, culture makes it very difficult for men to acknowledge and seek help for sexual dysfunction. Medical research has greatly advanced our understanding of the physiological basis of the two most common male sexual dysfunctions, rapid ejaculation (formerly termed premature ejaculation) and erectile dysfunction (formerly called impotence). Rapid ejaculation refers to involuntary male orgasm immediately or shortly following penetration. Erectile dysfunction refers to the inability to achieve or maintain an erection sufficient for penetration and male climax. There are medications that can reverse both conditions (SSRIs and sildenafil). There is also effective nonmedication treatment for both conditions.[1] Be aware that if there is no physiological basis for the problem, chances are that there is a relationship issue rather than some deep shameful defect in your individual psyche or masculinity. A family physician or urologist who specializes in sexuality is a good starting place to seek help for male sexual dysfunction.

Relax

My final sex tip is to try to relax about firing up the passion in your relationship. Have fun, be optimistic, expect to feel awkward at first, and give yourself permission to make mistakes. Don't view the sexual blahs as a nail in need of a hammer. There isn't a quick fix, and the only lasting change will be the gradual changes that come about as a result of small, continuous, and connected shifts in thinking, relating, and caring for one another's body and soul. Intimacy inside the bedroom nourishes and is nourished by intimacy outside the bedroom.

[1]See Bernie Zilbergeld, *The New Male Sexuality,* rev. ed. (New York: Bantam Doubleday Dell, 1999).

Appendix B: Sexual Dysfunction (Glossary of Terms)

The following terms are used by sex therapists, mental health professionals, and physicians to classify or describe diagnoses for sexual dysfunction. These terms are not set in stone, and there is considerable academic debate about how to classify sexual dysfunction. They are included here as a reference to help you identify issues that may be more serious than the sexual blahs. Understand that these are terms used in part for insurance purposes and not intended to place blame on either member of the couple.

In general, terms for sexual dysfunction are inclusive, and you may conclude that you have a "condition" when in fact you have an issue related to the diagnosis. In virtually every diagnostic classification, the problem described must cause "marked distress or interpersonal difficulty."[1] This is a subjective assessment best made by an experienced clinician. The other key aspect of diagnosis is that the problem must be persistent or recurrent. Beware the tendency to overdiagnose oneself, since psychological and sexual issues fall along a broad spectrum, and diagnosis is much more complex than healthy-versus-sick. Even when a definitive diagnosis is appropriate, sexual dysfunctions often reflect issues within the couple rather than within either spouse.

[1]Diagnostic and Statistical Manual of Mental Disorders, Text Revision (DSM-IV-TR) (Washington, D.C.: American Psychiatric Association, 2000).

Finally, be aware that the history of medicine is littered with conditions that once were attributed to mental conditions until their physical basis was appreciated. Noted examples include peptic ulcers, menstrual cramps, panic attacks, and epilepsy. Most recently, the introduction of a prescription medication for erectile dysfunction (Viagra) has revolutionized how physicians understand "impotence," just as antidepressants have changed how we understand clinical depression. However, neither a purely biological or purely psychological model is likely to prevail. The causes, like the solutions, will almost certainly prove to include a complex blend of hormones, anatomy, emotions, and relationships.

Hypoactive sexual desire disorder: Absent or constricted interest in sexual activity or sexual fantasies, often in an individual with intact physiological sexual arousal and orgasm. Examples may include low sex drive due to clinical depression, hormone deficiency, or severe marital dissatisfaction. A critical diagnostic issue is whether one member truly has low desire, whether he or she is mismatched with a partner with a higher sex drive, or if the other partner has an especially high sex drive.

Sexual aversion disorder: Unlike the reluctant sexual partner who experiences hypoactive sexual desire, an individual with sexual aversion disorder actively avoids sexual contact due to pronounced distaste for sex. He or she feels repulsed or anxious about the idea of sexual contact. An important diagnostic distinction should be made between Post-traumatic Stress Disorder, in which sexual aversion is attributable to prior sexual assault or abuse.

Female Sexual Arousal Disorder (FSAD): Arousal disorders in women are characterized by inadequate lubrication and swelling in response to escalating sexual arousal, although what the individual and her partner notice is dryness and secondary pain due to inadequate lubrication. This may be caused by breast-feeding or as a result of menopause or any physical condition that causes reduced blood flow to the pelvis, including some medications. Anxiety is another common cause of arousal disorder.

Male erectile disorder (also called erectile dysfunction): Formerly known as impotence, erectile disorder refers to the inability to achieve or maintain an erect penis sufficient to complete sexual intercourse. Any compromise of blood flow to the pelvis (which can result from smoking, high blood pressure, diabetes, medications, or vascular disease) can cause erectile dysfunction, which is also sometimes attributable to aging. As with women, anxiety may be the underlying cause.

Orgasmic disorders: Male and female orgasmic disorders are defined as the absence of or marked difficulty achieving sexual climax following "appropriate" sexual stimulation. Many clinicians prefer the term "preorgasmic" for women who have not yet achieved an orgasm, emphasizing that with appropriate experience and stimulation, most if not all previously nonorgasmic women can become orgasmic. Male orgasmic disorder during intercourse may be called "retarded ejaculation" or "male coital anorgasmia." There is considerable debate about whether an individual with normal physiology and anatomy is truly primarily nonorgasmic, since many apparently anorgasmic individuals are only situationally unable to climax, and numerous physical conditions cause secondary absence of orgasm (anorgasmia). Noted physical culprits include the SSRI antidepressants, including Celexa, Effexor, Luvox, Paxil, Prozac, and Zoloft, as well as alcohol abuse. Individuals with acquired (i.e., new onset) orgasmic disorders should be assumed to have a medical condition causing anorgasmia until proven otherwise.

Premature ejaculation (PE, also called rapid ejaculation): Rapid ejaculation that immediately follows penetration, before the man wishes to climax. Some clinicians use one minute as a standard, although there is considerable disagreement about the term (for example, adolescent males typically climax very quickly normatively). Cultural ideals about "real men" maintaining erections of mythical durations contribute to the controversy, as does the need to consider the partner's satisfaction. The term may be most useful for men who have never acquired ejaculatory delay or control, or those who have lost the ability to do so after previously satisfactory function. Premature ejaculation is the most common male sexual dysfunction. Anxiety about PE is a contributing factor and potential etiology.

Dyspareunia: This refers to painful intercourse (pain in the genitals or pelvis) and is considered by many clinicians to be better conceptualized as a pain problem rather than a sexual problem, in part because women with dyspareunia typically also experience pain upon gynecological examination, insertion of a tampon, etc. Current best-practice approaches to dyspareunia emphasize a multifaceted etiology and treatment model that recognizes the complex interaction of physical as well as emotional components. Vulvar vestibulitis and vulvar-vaginal atrophy associated with menopause may cause dyspareunia, as well as other gynecological conditions.

Vaginismus: Defined as involuntary muscle spasm of the vaginal muscles that prohibits sexual intercourse, vaginismus can be difficult to distinguish from dyspareunia. Some experts feel that vaginismus is a conditioned response to vulvar-vaginal pain, rather than a distinct entity. Since penetration is necessary for most reproduction, the rare mother who develops acquired (new-onset) vaginismus should be assumed to have an identifiable cause, such as sexual trauma or an underlying medical condition.

Resources

Ackerman, Diane. *A Natural History of the Senses.* New York: Vintage, 1991.

Barbach, Lonnie Garfield. *For Yourself: The Fulfillment of Female Sexuality,* rev. ed. New York: Signet, 2000.

———. ed. *The Erotic Edge: Erotica for Couples.* New York, Plume, 1996.

Basco, Monica Ramirez. *Never Good Enough: Freeing Yourself from the Chains of Perfectionism.* New York: Free Press, 1999.

Berman, Jennifer, Laura Berman, with Elisabeth Bumiller. *For Women Only: A Revolutionary Guide to Overcoming Sexual Dysfunction and Reclaiming Your Life.* New York: Henry Holt, 2001.

Breathnach, Sarah Ban. *Simple Abundance: A Daybook of Comfort and Joy.* New York: Warner, 1995.

Bright, Susie, ed. *The Best American Erotica 2001.* New York: Touchstone, 2001.

———. *Herotica 1: A Collection of Women's Erotic Fiction.* San Francisco: Down There Press, 1998.

Daniluk, Judith C. *Women's Sexuality Across the Lifespan: Challenging Myths, Creating Means.* New York: Guilford Press, 1998.

Domar, Alice, and Henry Dreher. *Self-Nurture: Learning to Care for Yourself as Effectively as You Care for Everyone Else.* New York: Penguin, 2001.

Friday, Nancy. *My Secret Garden: Women's Sexual Fantasies,* 25th ed. New York: Pocket, 1998.

Gottman, John M., and Nan Silver. *The Seven Principles for Making Marriage Work.* New York: Three Rivers Press, 2000.

Heiman, Julia R., and Joseph Lopiccolo. *Becoming Orgasmic: A Sexual and Personal Growth Program for Women,* rev. ed. New York: Fireside, 1988.

Jones, Richard Glyn, and A. Susan Williams, eds. *The Penguin Book of Erotic Stories by Women.* New York: Penguin, 1996.

Kenison, Katrina. *Mitten Strings for God: Reflections for Mothers in a Hurry.* New York: Warner, 2000.

Lerner, Harriet. *The Mother Dance: What Children Do to Your Life.* New York: HarperCollins, 1999.

Lloyd, Joan Elizabeth. *52 Saturday Nights: Heat Up Your Sex Life Even More with a Year of Creative Lovemaking.* New York: Warner, 2000.

Maltz, Wendy, and Suzie Boss. *Private Thoughts: Exploring the Power of Women's Sexual Fantasies.* New York: New World Library, 2001.

McGraw, Phillip C. *Relationship Rescue.* New York: Hyperion, 2000.

Michael, Robert T., John H. Gagnon, Edward O. Laumann, and Gina Kolata. *Sex in America: A Definitive Survey.* New York: Warner Books, 1995.

Mohanraj, Mary Anne, ed. *Aqua Erotica: 18 Stories for a Steamy Bath.* New York: Three Rivers Press, 2000.

Placksin, Sally. *Mothering the New Mother: Women's Feelings and Needs After Childbirth, a Support and Resource Guide.* New York: Newmarket Press, 2000.

Rako, Susan. *The Hormone of Desire: The Truth About Testosterone, Sexuality and Menopause.* New York: Three Rivers Press, 1999.

Reichman, Judith. *I'm Not in the Mood: What Every Woman Should Know About Improving Her Libido.* New York: Morrow, 1998.

Renshaw, Domeena. *Seven Weeks to Better Sex.* New York: Dell, 1995.

Rosenfeld, Alvin, and Nicole Wise. *Hyper-Parenting: Are You Hurting Your Child by Trying Too Hard?* New York: St. Martin's Press, 2000.

Semans, Anne, and Cathy Winks. *The Woman's Guide to Sex on the Web.* San Francisco: HarperSanFrancisco, 1999.

Sudo, Philip Toshio. *Zen Sex: The Way of Making Love.* San Francisco: HarperSanFrancisco, 2000.

Thornton, Laura, Jan Sturtevant, and Amber Coverdale Sumrall, eds. *Touching Fire: Erotic Writings by Women.* New York: Carroll & Graf, 1989.

Webb, Michael, *The RoMANtic's Guide: Hundreds of Creative Tips for a Lifetime of Love.* New York: Hyperion, 2000.

Zilbergeld, Bernie. *The New Male Sexuality,* rev. ed. New York: Doubleday Dell, 1999.

Web Sites*

See page 186 for tips on mom-friendly erotic web browsing.

www.bodypositive.com
www.cleansheets.com
www.erotica-readers.com
www.goaskalice.columbia.edu
www.hipmama.com
www.ivillage.com
www.nerve.com
www.oxygen.com
www.redbook.women.com
www.salon.com/sex/index.html
www.scarletletters.com
www.susiebright.com

Retail Web Sites

www.babeland.com
www.royalle.com
www.drugstore.com
www.evesgarden.com
www.goodvibes.com
www.redenvelope.com

Acknowledgments

My heartfelt thanks to Anne Edelstein, Marah Stets, Trish Todd, and Tracy Schneider, who provided invigorating and much-appreciated advocacy and support of this book from its infancy.

I am profoundly grateful to Doris Cooper, my editor, for her magic. Your perceptive, thoughtful, kind, and detailed attention has been invaluable.

I am also indebted to the fellow moms who generously read and commented on earlier drafts. Thanks especially to Debra Abrahamson, Jill Baskin, Maryla Blum, and Lisa Groves.

A special thanks to Charles Adamczyk, M.D., for sharing his wise and caring expertise as an obstetrician-gynecologist.